Springer Series on Geriatric Nursing

Mathy D. Mezey, RN, EdD, FAAN, Series Editor
New York University Division of Nursing

Advisory Board: Margaret Dimond, PhD, RN, FAAN; Steven H. Ferris, PhD; Terry Fulmer, RN, PhD, FAAN; Linda Kaeser, PhD, RN, ACSW, FAAN; Virgene Kayser-Jones, PhD, RN, FAAN; Eugenia Siegler, MD; Neville E. Strumpf, PhD, RN, FAAN; May Wykle, PhD, RN, FAAN; Mary K. Walker, PhD, RN, FAAN

2004   **Care of Gastrointestinal Problems in the Older Adult**
Sue E. Meiner, EdD, APRN, BC, GNP

2003   **Geriatric Nursing Protocols for Best Practice, 2nd ed.**
Mathy D. Mezey, EdD, RN, FAAN, Terry Fulmer, PhD, RN, FAAN, Ivo Abraham, PhD, RN, FAAN, De Anne Zwicker, Managing Editor, MA, APRN, BC

2002   **Care of Arthritis in the Older Adult**
Ann Schmidt Luggen, PhD, RN, MSN, CS, BC-ARNP, and Sue E. Meiner, EdD, APRN, BC, GNP

2002   **Prostate Cancer: Nursing Assessment, Management, and Care**
Meredith Wallace, PhD, RN, CS-ANP, and Lorrie L. Powel, PhD, RN

2002   **Bathing Without a Battle: Personal Care of Individuals With Dementia**
Ann Louise Barrick, PhD, Joanne Rader, RN, MN, FAAN, Beverly Hoeffer, DNSc, RN, FAAN, and Philip D. Sloane, MD, MPH

2001   **Critical Care Nursing of the Elderly, Second Edition**
Terry Fulmer, PhD, RN, FAAN, Marquis D. Foreman, PhD, RN, FAAN, Mary Walker, PhD, RN, FAAN, and Kristen S. Montgomery, PhD, RNC, IBCLC

1999   **Geriatric Nursing Protocols for Best Practice**
Ivo Abraham, PhD, RN, FAAN, Melissa M. Bottrell, MPH, Terry T. Fulmer, PhD, RN, FAAN, and Mathy D. Mezey, EdD, RN, FAAN

1998   **Home Care for Older Adults: A Guide for Families and Other Caregivers—Text and Instructor's Manual/Lesson Plan**
Mary Ann Rosswurm, EdD, RN, CS, FAAN

1998   **Restraint-Free Care: Individualized Approaches for Frail Elders**
Neville E. Strumpf, PhD, RN, C, FAAN, Joanne Patterson Robinson, PhD, RN, Joan Stockman Wagner, MSN, CRNP, and Lois K. Evans, DNSc, RN, FAAN

1996   **Gerontology Review Guide for Nurses**
Elizabeth Chapman Shaid, RN, MSN, CRNP, and Kay Huber, DEd, RN, CRNP

1995   **Strengthening Geriatric Nursing Education**
Terry T. Fulmer, RN, PhD, FAAN, and Marianne Matzo, PhD, RN, CS

1994   **Nurse-Physician Collaboration: Care of Adults and the Elderly**
Eugenia L. Siegler, MD, and Fay W. Whitney, PhD, RN, FAAN

1993   **Health Assessment of the Older Individual, Second Edition**
Mathy D. Mezey, RN, EdD, FAAN, Louise H. Rauckhorst, RNC, ANP, EdD, and Shirlee Ann Stokes, RN, EdD, FAAN

1992   **Critical Care Nursing of the Elderly**
Terry T. Fulmer, RN, PhD, FAAN, and Mary K. Walker, PhD, RN, FAAN

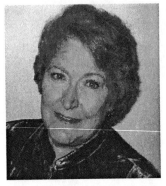

Sue E. Meiner, EdD, APRN, BC, GNP, is an Assistant Professor in the School of Nursing at the University of Nevada, Las Vegas, and a Gerontological Nurse Practitioner with HealthEssentials Home Care in Las Vegas. She received her BSN and MSN degrees at St. Louis University (Missouri), her EdD at Southern Illinois University at Edwardsville, and her GNP from Jewish Hospital College of Nursing and Allied Health at Washington University Medical Center in St. Louis, Missouri. She holds two national certifications from the American Nurses Credentialing Center. Dr. Meiner is certified as a Gerontological Clinical Nurse Specialist and as a Gerontological Nurse Practitioner. Prior to her current position, she was Project Director for an NIH and NIA grant at Washington University School of Medicine (St. Louis). Dr. Meiner has authored the book, *Nursing Documentation: Legal Focus Across Practice Settings.* She is co-author of several other books, including *Care of Arthritis in the Older Adult,* NGNA Core Curricula for both gerontological nurses and gerontological advanced practice nurses, and *Handbook for the Care of Older Adults with Cancer.* She is also the author of numerous book chapters and journal articles. Dr. Meiner held an elected political office in St. Louis County for five years in the 1980s and remains active in community service. For over 15 years, she has served nationally as an expert witness on nursing standards of care.

Care of Gastrointestinal Problems in the Older Adult

Sue E. Meiner, EdD, APRN, BC, GNP

Editor

 Springer Publishing Company

Springer Publishing Company, Inc.
536 Broadway
New York, NY 10012-3955

Acquisitions Editor: Ruth Chasek
Production Editor: Janice Stangel
Cover design by Joanne Honigman

04 05 06 07 08 / 5 4 3 2 1

Library of Congress Cataloging-in-Publication Data

Care of gastrointestinal problems in the older adult / Sue Meiner, editor.
    p. ; cm. — (Springer series on geriatric nursing)
    Includes bibliographical references and index.
    ISBN 0-8261-1865-8
    1. Geriatric gastroenterology. 2. Geriatric nursing. [DNLM: 1. Gastrointestinal Diseases—nursing—Aged. 2. Geriatric Nursing—methods. WY 156.5 C271 2004]
    I. Meiner, Sue. II. Series.
    RC802.4.A34C37 2004
    618.97'633—dc22   2004004159

Printed in the United States of America by Integrated Book Technology

I dedicate this book to my family, friends, and caring professionals in the fields of nursing, nursing education, and advanced practice nursing. I extend a very special thanks to Ruth Chasek, Nursing Editor with Springer Publishing Company, for her hours of support during the high, and sometimes low, road of writing and finishing a manuscript. And finally, in God I trust.

Contents

Contributors

Phyllis Atkinson, MSN, RN, CS, GN
St. Elizabeth Medical Center
Family Practice Center
Edgewood, Kentucky

Lori Candela, EdD, MSN, RN
Interim Associate Director
School of Nursing
University of Nevada, Las Vegas

Donna Sue Clarren, ND, MSN, RN
Assistant Professor
School of Nursing
University of Nevada, Las Vegas

Lynn Ferebee, MSN, RN, FNP
Family Nurse Practitioner
Student Health Center
University of Nevada, Las Vegas
Las Vegas, Nevada

Catherine Hill, MSN, RN, CS, ONC, CEN
Medicine Associates of North Texas
School of Nursing
University of Texas at Arlington

Susan Kowalski, PhD, MSN, RN
Associate Professor
School of Nursing
University of Nevada, Las Vegas

Ann Schmidt Luggen, PhD, MSN, APRN, GNP
Professor of Nursing
Northern Kentucky University
Highland Heights, Kentucky

Beverly Reno, MSN, RNC
Associate Professor of Nursing
Northern Kentucky University
Highland Heights, Kentucky

Barbara Resnick, PhD, CRNP, FAAN, FAANP
Associate Professor
University of Maryland School of Nursing
Baltimore, Maryland

Preface

As a gerontological nurse practitioner, I see many older adults with gastro-intestinal disorders that have been troubling them for decades. Even my personal experience with family and friends has brought home the prevalence of gastrointestinal problems in older adulthood.

This book was developed to provide greater information on a variety of gastrointestinal disorders and problems than can be found in general nursing textbooks. While the information in this book ranges from general to scientific, it is intended for use by a wide variety of nursing professionals from hospital nurses, to home care nurses, to nurse practitioners. Each clinician should choose the aspects of the text that are relevant to his or her practice. However, the overall content will add more specific knowledge to caring for the most common gastrointestinal problems of older adults.

Most of the chapters follow a pattern that includes discussion of a specific gastrointestinal problem followed by its cause, noted normal and abnormal physiology, nursing care with attention to nursing diagnoses, interventions, medications, and alternative therapies, where appropriate. Topics such as health promotion and quality of life issues were added as an essential part of any plan of care for older adults. Home management and self-care issues are addressed.

I hope that you will learn much from this book and will use the information to make the life of the older adults you care for more comfortable during their remaining life.

Sue E. Meiner, EdD, APRN, BC, GNP

–1–

Introduction and Demographic Data

Sue E. Meiner

Successful aging can have many different meanings. Freedom from illness and disease is a wishful thought as the life span progresses over many decades after the fifth decade of life. The aging process includes maturity in thinking, planning, acting, and evaluating the outcomes of decisions. It also means the aging of the human body. Some of the changes that occur with aging include declining function of some organs and body systems, which can produce illnesses and disease processes. While aging does not have to mean experiencing ill health, the changes in physiology associated with aging are often associated with illness and disease. Given patterns of decline may be in structure or function, whether from aging or disease or both, the decline may not be noticed until it reaches a level that is beyond the individual's ability to adapt. Successful aging includes successful adaptation to changes. When stress, in many forms, is placed on a body system, the older adult may not have the prolonged ability to adapt, thus leading to an inability of that body system to continue its normal function. When this occurs, illness or a disease process may begin. One system of the body that is vulnerable to illness and disease throughout the life span is the gastrointestinal (GI) system. However, the incidence of gastrointestinal (GI) disease increases with age, making the older adult the most sensitive to the broadest range of disorders.

Many GI tract disorders begin with a loss of appetite and nausea, with or without vomiting. Nausea is an ill-defined, unpleasant sensation that is often accompanied by pallor, sweating, and tachycardia. It can be followed by vomiting. This expulsive discharge of the contents of the stomach might or might not relieve the feeling of nausea. Continued nausea usually results in loss of appetite and potential weight loss. These examples are presented to demonstrate the human suffering that often accompanies GI disorders. More complicated GI conditions of older adults account for great personal expenditure for treatment, and a drain on the nation's economy (National Digestive Diseases Information Clearinghouse, 2002).

Every year approximately 62 million Americans are diagnosed with GI tract diseases (National Digestive Diseases Information Clearinghouse, 2002). Other than gastroenteritis and appendicitis, which are predominantly pediatric illnesses, and hemorrhoids, inflammatory bowel disease, and chronic liver disease, which are found predominantly among young and middle-aged people, the incidence and prevalence of GI disorders from the oral cavity to the anus are seen more frequently with advancing age. Digestive diseases may be acute and self-limiting, chronic and debilitating, or sudden and devastating.

The cause and progression of many GI tract diseases are unknown, but a family history of similar symptoms or even a diagnosis of the same disease in another family member is a frequent finding. Additional factors that are associated with patterns of gastrointestinal tract symptoms may include prolonged stress, fatigue, food choices, smoking, and alcohol abuse. Alcohol abuse is the highest risk factor for GI diseases, particularly for esophageal, colorectal, and liver cancers (National Digestive Diseases Information Clearinghouse, 2002).

Women are more likely than men to report a GI problem to their primary care providers. The reason for this is assumed to be the frequency of women's visits to health care professionals compared with the number of visits made by men (National Digestive Diseases Information Clearinghouse, 2002).

Some general disorders of the upper GI tract pose difficulties for older adults. These include odynophagia, dyspepsia, dysphagia, hiatal hernia, regurgitation, pyrosis, and/or esophagitis. Most hiatal hernias are caused by a physical abnormality that may be present at birth. These disorders will be discussed in Chapter 2. Another major problem for older adults is gastroesophageal reflux disease, more commonly referred to as GERD. Nearly one-third of the American population is affected with symptoms of GERD. This disease will be discussed in Chapter 3.

Problems with the stomach can span motor dysfunctions, ulcers, bacterial or viral infections, and vitamin deficiencies. Motor dysfunctions relate to rapid emptying disorders to delayed emptying conditions. These will be presented in Chapter 4. Peptic ulcer disease is estimated to affect 4.5 million people in the United States. This disease is responsible for substantial human suffering and a large economic burden. The various illnesses caused by ulcers, especially those resulting from infection with Helicobacter pylori will be discussed in Chapter 5. Food-borne illness results from eating food contaminated with bacteria, viruses, parasites, and other pathogens. These illnesses can range from an upset stomach to more severe symptoms that can lead to dehydration and even death in more vulnerable people. Other bacterial diseases, and infections caused by viruses and parasites will be presented in Chapter 6. The role of deficiencies from vitamin B_{12} and folic acid (folate) are important to add to any discussion of GI illnesses. Chapter 7 will present information on vitamin B_{12} and folate deficiencies.

Predominant cancers of the GI tract are oropharyngeal, esophageal, stomach, gallbladder, pancreatic, liver, small intestine, colon, and rectal. Chapter 8 will provide information on these cancers, statistics on their incidence and prevalence, and care issues.

Nutrition is essential to life and the GI tract is the organ system that accepts, processes, and provides benefit to the body from the foods that are eaten. While basic nutrition needs to be understood, specialty diets and food preparation issues are an integral part of treating GI disorders, illnesses, and diseases. Chapter 9 will provide information on general nutrition and the special nutritional needs of older adults.

Diseases, disorders, and illnesses of the lower GI tract will cover specific concerns related to irritable bowel syndrome (IBS), diverticular disease, constipation, noninfectious diarrhea, hemorrhoids, and problems of the rectum and anus. Irritable bowel is a common functional disorder of the intestines with an unknown cause. The term "functional" refers to a disorder with symptoms of disease but without findings on diagnostic testing. This will be explained in Chapter 10.

Diverticula are pouchings, approximately the size of large peas, formed in the intestinal walls. The more common location is in the large intestine or colon. Diverticulosis is very common, especially in older adults. It is estimated that nearly half of all persons over the age of 60 have diverticulosis. Diverticulitis is characterized by inflammation and subsequent infection of one or more diverticuli. However, when diverticulitis becomes complicated, abscesses, bowel obstruction, or fistulae can occur.

Constipation and noninfectious diarrhea are problems that are common among older adults. Constipation is the passage of small amounts of hard, dry stools, usually fewer than three times a week. The feeling of being bloated, accompanied by sluggish behavior and general discomfort are usual when constipation is present. Noninfectious diarrhea, which is the passing of loose, watery stools occurring more than three times in one day is less common than constipation in the older adult, but can lead to dehydration or electrolyte disturbances, and needs immediate treatment. Constipation and noninfectious diarrhea will be presented in Chapter 12.

Hemorrhoids are redundant mucosa, venous and arterial plexuses, smooth muscle, and connective tissue in the submucosa of the anal canal. Hemorrhoids are not varicose veins of the rectum. After age 50, hemorrhoids are common in approximately 75% of older adults. Hemorrhoids, rectal prolapse, proctitis, and anal disorders are presented in Chapter 13.

The symptoms of many GI diseases are subtle, yet complex, and can be difficult to diagnose early in an illness. Many disorders have similar symptoms and differentiating the specific symptoms of a single disease often takes time and several visits to the health care professional. Diagnostic tests can include blood tests, an upper, lower, or combined GI series of radiographs, an abdominal ultrasound, and an endoscopic examination of the esophagus, stomach, small intestine, colon, or rectum. If answers are still pending, a CT scan or an MRI can reveal physiologic information that can assist in making a diagnosis.

Treatment options include dietary changes, physical activity, watchful waiting, and prescription or over-the-counter medications as recommended by a primary care provider.

According to the National Institutes of Health, digestive diseases cost nearly $107 billion in direct health care expenditures. These illnesses result in approximately 200 million sick days, 50 million visits to physicians, 16.9 million days lost from school, and 10 million hospitalizations. Nearly 200,000 deaths per year are attributable to GI diseases (National Digestive Diseases Information Clearinghouse, 2002).

When the yearly costs of each of the major GI diseases are calculated, the five most expensive are diarrheal infections ($4.7 billion); gallbladder disease and colorectal cancer ($4.5 billion); liver disease ($3.2 billion); and peptic ulcer disease ($2.5 billion). Of the acute, noncancerous GI medical conditions reported (440 million) in the United States annually, over 22 million are for acute GI conditions, with 11 million from gastroenteritis. Another six million cases are related to indigestion, nausea, and vomiting (National Digestive Disease Information Clearinghouse, 2002).

Deaths due to cancers of the GI tract total 117,000 deaths annually. Of the noncancerous GI disease deaths each year, the single largest killer is chronic liver disease which accounts for 36% (National Digestive Diseases Information Clearinghouse, 2002).

Diseases of the GI tract have a massive influence on health and the health care system in the United States. New technologies and new drugs have revolutionized the comprehension and treatment of peptic ulcer disease and GERD. The success of future research will, optimistically, continue to reduce the economic and health care costs related to diagnosing and treating digestive diseases.

REFERENCES

National Digestive Disease Information Clearinghouse (2002). Overview of digestive diseases, retrieved from *www.niddk.nih.gov/health/digest/pubs/overview.htm*

—2—

General Disorders of the Upper Gastrointestinal System

Beverly Anderson Reno

The upper gastrointestinal (GI) system is important in the breakdown and digestion of food. Digestion occurs through the mastication of food, and the production of mucus and enzymes, which further break down carbohydrates. Once in the esophagus the bolus of food propels into the stomach. A primary function of the lower esophageal sphincter is to prevent the gastric contents from back flowing backwards into the esophagus.

The stomach is a food reservoir and has a secretory function. There are hormones (gastrin) which stimulate the secretion of hydrochloric acid by the parietal cells. The parietal cells are also responsible for the production of the intrinsic and extrinsic factors that enhance the absorption of vitamin B_{12}. The first part of the small intestine is also included because of the continual breakdown of food into nutrients for the body. Older adults have a decrease in gastric motility, and a decrease in the gag and swallowing reflexes. The older adult is also at risk for a decrease in the tone of the esophageal sphincter.

The following physiological factors are either directly involved in the development of GERD (gastroesophageal reflux) or are the result of GERD.

ODYNOPHAGIA

This is termed painful swallowing and can often be the result of GERD. It is most common in immunocompromised clients. It also may be indicative of an esophageal stricture.

Etiology

The most common cause of odynophagia is infectious esophagitis. The client experiences severe substernal chest pain due to esophageal spasms. The pain can be excruciating and can last for several hours.

Pathology

Infectious esophagitis in the older adult is most often a result of Candida albicans, cytomegalovirus, or herpes simplex virus. It can also be the result of chemical burns or pill related. The stricture may be the result of a tumor or growth around the esophagus.

General Nursing Care

1. Complete a nursing history and assessment of the upper GI system.
2. Complete a pain assessment according to guidelines of location, radiation, what relieves, what exacerbates, and duration (use the pain scale for documentation).
3. Provide for comfort measures through pain management.
4. Provide for emotional support by giving reassurance when episodes of pain occur.
5. Teach client about diagnostic tests such as barium swallow and endoscopy to relieve anxiety.

Nursing Diagnoses

1. Pain related to esophageal spasms secondary to infection
2. Fear related to tests being administered
3. Anxiety related to unknown diagnosis

Interventions, Treatments, Alternative Treatments

1. Teach client and family about diet changes, i.e., avoid carbonated and caffeinated beverages. Eliminate highly spiced and seasoned foods from diet, (grilled and smoked).
2. Administer proton pump inhibitors such as omeprazole (Prilosec), which blocks acid production in the stomach, and lansoprazole (Prevacid), which suppresses gastric acid secretion in the stomach. Histamine receptor antagonists like ranitidine (Zantac) and famotidine (Pepcid), which inhibit gastric acid secretion.
3. Monitor effectiveness of drug therapy.

Health Promotion and Quality of Life Issues

1. Teach client and family about the adverse effects of alcohol, smoking and drug use.
2. Assess client's coping skills. If maladaptive, teach alternative coping skills and assist the client in identifying more effective ways to swallow food and fluids.
3. Support client in making own decisions on what their expectations are in relation to quality of life issues.

Home Management and Self-Care Issues

1. Assess support systems: family, friends, neighborhood, and faith community.
2. Assess knowledge of community support services available.
3. Assess for transportation needs.
4. Assess for financial resources.
5. Assess for ability to manage within the home.
6. Refer to home health agency if appropriate.
7. Teach client and family to avoid over-the-counter drugs (OTC) when taking prescribed drugs.
8. Utilize effective coping skills during stressful situations.

Follow-up Care

1. Stress the importance to family and client of follow-up care with their health care provider.

DYSPEPSIA

Dyspepsia is referred to as pyrosis, heartburn, or indigestion. It is a classic symptom of GERD. Dyspepsia is a common problem but rarely considered serious unless other symptomatology occurs. Nonulcerative dyspepsia is often referred to as a functional disorder. There is a 15–20% incidence in adults 45 years and older.

Etiology

The exact cause is unknown and the symptoms are nonspecific to any one disease. Precipitating factors include diet high in fatty, spicy, and highly seasoned foods, overeating, caffeine intake, smoking, and medications. All of these foods may precipitate the irritation of the esophagus. The client often experiences mild to severe pain. The pain is described as burning and may be referred to as back pain. In severe pain, it may be described as radiating to jaw or neck and can mimic angina (Lyder, 1998).

Pathology

When acid refluxes into the esophagus, a burning sensation is present posterior to the breastbone and is called heartburn.

General Nursing Care

1. Complete a nursing history and physical exam of the upper GI system.
2. Complete a dietary history.
3. Elicit a complete pain history according to guidelines (see above)
4. Inform client of tests to be performed, purpose of tests, and preparation for the tests.

Nursing Diagnoses

1. Knowledge deficit related to dietary needs and restrictions.
2. Pain related to esophageal irritation.

Interventions, Treatments, Alternative Treatments

1. Teach client to avoid the recumbent and bending over positions, as the pain usually worsens. Maintain an upright position.
2. Instruct to drink fluids to assist in relieving the pain.
3. Administer antacids (Maalox, Mylanta, Rolaids, and TUMS).
4. Administer acid blockers such as Zantac (ranitidine), Pepcid (famotidine), Axid (nizsatidine), and Tagamet (cimetidine). Other drugs given are proton pump inhibitors, prokinetics, antispasmodics, and low-dose antidepressants.
5. Teach client to chew food slowly and completely
6. Avoid eating large meals; eat several small meals throughout the day.

Health Promotion and Quality of Life Issues

1. Teach client about lifestyle changes that will reduce intra-abdominal pressure, which reduces the incidence of dyspepsia (sleep with head of bed elevated). Limit straining, lifting, pulling, or pushing.
2. Identify effective coping skills and stressors.
3. Teach client to utilize effective coping skills such as walking, listening to music, and imagery with progressive relaxation of muscles. Exercise in early evening.
4. Suggest meals be leisurely: no conflicts and a calm environment may decrease the occurrences of stress-related dyspepsia.

Home Management and Self-Care Issues

1. Assess support systems: family, friends, neighborhood, and faith community.
2. Assess knowledge of community support services available.
3. Assess for transportation needs.
4. Assess for financial resources.
5. Assess for ability to manage within the home.
6. Refer to home health agency if appropriate.
7. Teach client when to call their health care provider such as increase in symptoms of dyspepsia (heartburn, indigestion).
8. Instruct client to notify health care provider if vomiting of blood or passing of bloody stools occurs, profuse sweating with pain, chest pain or pattern of dyspepsia significantly changes.

9. Refrain from activities that result in excessive swallowing of air such as smoking, drinking carbonated beverages, and chewing gum.

Follow-up Care

1. Stress the importance of follow-up care with the client's health care provider.

DYSPHAGIA

Dysphagia is a result of a malfunction in the swallowing process. It is experienced as difficulty in swallowing. There is a sequence of events in the swallowing process. Muscular contractions and relaxation can be categorized into three phases the oral, oropharyngeal, and esophageal. Dysphagia can be termed either "oropharyngeal" or "esophageal." Oropharyngeal dysphagia occurs before the bolus of food reaches the upper esophagus and esophageal results from problems after the bolus of food reaches the esophagus. Dysphagia occurs with the first ingestion of food. It should not be progressive or constant (Mayo Clinic, 2002).

Etiology

In older adults, central nervous system disorders including dementias, strokes, or Alzheimer's usually result in oropharyngeal dysphagia. The most common type of dysphagia is esophageal. Common causes are gastric motility disorders (achalasia), tumors, and reflux esophagitis. Also in older adults, there is a reduction in salivation, a decrease in muscle strength for mastication, and loss of teeth, which all can increase the risk of dysphagia. Clients usually present with complaints of "feeling something stuck" in their throat, or pain in the throat or chest, which may suggest spasms of the esophagus or GERD (National Guideline Clearinghouse, 1999).

Pathology

Oropharyngeal dysphagia is the result of weakened muscles in the throat, which may cause choking and coughing when attempting to swallow.

Esophageal dysphagia may be directly related to peptic strictures, tumors, diverticulae, psychological factors, pill ingestion, and reflux esophagitis.

General Nursing Care

1. Complete a comprehensive upper GI exam.
2. Evaluate swallowing difficulties to determine if only at beginning of meal vs. progressive and persistent. Questions to ask: Do you have difficulty swallowing solids, liquids, or both? Does choking occur when eating or drinking? Do you have pain with swallowing? Is indigestion a problem?
3. Do you have a decrease in salivation?
4. Complete a nutritional assessment.
5. Consult with a speech therapist about a swallowing evaluation.
6. Inform client of tests (barium swallow, endoscopy, and manometry), purpose of tests, and preparation for the tests (Ignaatavius & Workman, 2002).

Nursing Diagnoses

1. High risk for injury, aspiration related to weakened throat muscles.
2. High risk for alterations in nutrition related to progressive dysphagia.
3. Knowledge deficit related to treatment regimen.

Interventions, Treatments, Alternative Treatments

1. Teach client to be in sitting position when eating.
2. Provide a sucker to enhance tongue strength.
3. Provide for thickened liquids. Consult with dietician about appropriate thickness (honey, pudding, etc.).
4. Prepare for surgery if client is candidate for esophageal dilation.
5. Assist client with diet selections to include semisoft foods if decreased saliva is problem for swallowing.
6. Monitor for signs and symptoms of aspiration.
7. Administer prescribed medications on scheduled times. Antireflux drugs such as proton pump inhibitors, nitrates (esophageal spasms), anticholinergics (see meds in Dyspepsia).

Health Promotion and Quality of Life Issues

1. Teach client about lifestyle changes that will increase quality of life.
2. Assess for leisure activities and encourage involvement in social activities.
3. Assess if patient has living will and discuss client's options if emergency occurs.
4. Assess clients coping skills and teach methods to reduce stress (relaxation, music, deep breathing, having a special friend).

Home Management and Self-Care Issues

1. Assess support systems: family, friends, neighborhood, and faith community.
2. Assess knowledge of community support services available.
3. Assess for transportation needs.
4. Assess for financial resources.
5. Assess for ability to manage within the home.
6. Refer to home health agency if appropriate.
7. Instruct family and client on lifesaving measures if choking episode occurs.
8. If appropriate, teach the family how to help the client with the "chin tuck." This is done by positioning the head forward and the chin back into the neck before swallowing.
9. Collaborate with speech therapist in teaching the family and client how to perform swallowing exercises. These can include using thickened liquids and concentrating on swallowing each spoonful of food while using the chin tuck. Avoiding a dry mouth is essential to the success of home management of dysphagia. Speech therapy can provide a wide variety of exercises specifically for each client's needs.
10. Teach the family how to prepare thickened liquids and semisoft food if appropriate.
11. Encourage family to allow client to be independent in ADLs (activities of daily living).
12. Teach family the importance of monitoring food and liquid intake (Ignaatavius & Workman, 2002).

Follow-up Care

1. Stress the importance to family and client of follow-up care with their client health care provider.

HIATAL HERNIA

Commonly referred to as a diaphragmatic hernia, it forms at the small opening in the diaphragm. This opening is known as the hiatus of the diaphragm. The hernia is the protrusion of the fundus of the stomach into the diaphragmatic hiatus.

Etiology

The development of a hiatal hernia occurs because of a weakened esophageal muscle surrounding the diaphragmatic opening. This weakness allows the stomach fundus to protrude through the diaphragm into the thoracic cavity. Constant pressure such as lifting heavy articles, Valsalva maneuver (holding the breath and tightening abdominal muscles), continuous vomiting, or coughing can put undue stress on the diaphragmatic opening again allowing the stomach to protrude into the thoracic cavity. Key manifestations of hernias are heartburn, regurgitation, belching, chest pain, feelings of fullness or breathlessness after eating, and dysphagia (CHID Digestive Diseases, 1999).

Pathology

There are two types of hernias. The sliding hernia is the most common in persons over the age of 50, and accounts for 90% of all diagnosed hernias. The prevalence of this type of hernia increases with age. In fact, there is a 60% occurrence in persons over the age of 60. This hernia moves in and out of the thorax in direct relation to positions of pressure on the diaphragm such as lying flat, and increases in intra-abdominal pressure. A major complication is the development of gastroesophageal reflux. When the hiatal hernia pushes the esophageal sphincter above the diaphragm, the pressure on the sphincter is reduced which then results in the backflow of stomach secretions into the esophagus.

The second type of hernia is a rolling hernia (para-esophageal). This hernia results in not only the fundus of the stomach but also the curvature to roll through the esophageal hiatus into the thorax and align beside the esophagus. The major concerns are strangulation, obstruction, and volvulus.

General Nursing Care

1. Inform client of tests (barium swallow, X-ray, and endoscopy).
2. Assess for comfort needs and administer pain medication as appropriate.
3. Medically manage sliding hernias.
4. Prepare clients with paraesophageal hernias for possible Nissen anti-reflux surgical repair. Indications are strangulation, volvulus, and obstruction.

Nursing Diagnoses

1. Alteration in comfort/pain related to esophageal reflux.
2. Alteration in nutrition: less than body requirement related to feelings of fullness and breathlessness with eating.
3. Knowledge deficit related to disease process.

Interventions, Treatment, Alternative Treatments

1. Administer antacids (Mylanta, Maalox, Tums) according to proto-col. Administer histamine receptor blockers: cimetidine (Tagamet), ranitidine (Zantac), and famotidine (Pepcid) and proton pump in-hibitors (PPIs): lansoprazole (Prevacid) and omeprazole (Prilosec).
2. Instruct client to take medications before meals, or if taken when symptoms occur, expect at least 30 minutes for effect.
3. Inform client of side effects of drugs: dry mouth, dizziness, constipa-tion all may occur with antacids and histamine blockers. Diarrhea, headache, and stomach and abdominal pain can occur with proton pump inhibitors.
4. Teach client preparation for diagnostic tests.
5. Assess for bowel strangulation and obstruction.

6. Teach client to remain in upright position after eating for at least 3 hours before resting or retiring for the night. Raise head of bed 30–45 degrees or sleep on 2–3 pillows to prevent increase in abdominal pressure.
7. Teach client to avoid snacking before bedtime, this increases acid formation.
8. Avoid straining with bowel movements and avoid activities which require stooping and bending (Ignaatavius & Workman, 2002).

Health Promotion and Quality of Life Issues

1. Teach client about lifestyle changes that will enhance quality of life by reducing pain and discomfort from hernia.
2. Identify effective coping skills that follow the nursing interventions and give positive feedback.
3. Identify ineffective coping skills, such as smoking, drinking, and use of recreational drugs as a response to stressors.

Home Management and Self-Care Issues

1. Assess support systems: family, friends, neighborhood, and faith community.
2. Assess knowledge of community support services available.
3. Assess for transportation needs.
4. Assess for financial resources.
5. Assess for ability to manage within the home.
6. Refer to home health agency if appropriate.
7. Teach client to lose weight. Being overweight is the single most important contributing factor in causing problems with hernias.

Follow-up Care

1. Stress the importance to family and client about follow-up care with their health care provider.

REGURGITATION

Regurgitation is related to neither eructation (belching) nor nausea and vomiting. It is a common symptom of gastroesophageal reflux (GERD).

Etiology/Pathology

Regurgitation is failure of the lower esophageal sphincter (LES) to close. It can be related to a lower pressure in the thorax, which directly affects the LES closure. The client experiences warm fluid flowing upward into the esophagus and mouth. These regurgitated gastric contents may result in a bitter taste in the mouth.

General Nursing Care

1. Provide for emotional support by giving reassurance when episodes of dysphagia, choking, or chest pain occur.
2. Provide for comfort measures through pain management (Ignaatavius & Workman, 2002).

Nursing Diagnoses

1. Alteration in comfort related to regurgitation of gastric fluids.
2. Anxiety related to undiagnosed chest pain.
3. Social isolation related to choking episodes.
4. High risk for injury: aspiration related to backflow of gastric fluids.

Interventions, Treatments, Alternative Treatments

1. Teach client foods to avoid highly seasoned, fatty foods.
2. Teach client to remain in upright position during and after eating.
3. Assess lung sounds for crackles, which would indicate chemical aspiration.
4. Assess for presence of bronchitis in clients with long-standing regurgitation problems, due to the association of aspiration and irritation to the bronchi.
5. Encourage client to maintain social outings, remembering to eat slowly and avoid problem foods.

Health Promotion and Quality of Life Issues/Home Management and Self-Care Issues

1. Encourage client to avoid alcohol, smoking, and use of recreational drugs, spicy foods, fatty foods, and large meals.

2. Teach client to administer medications as directed and avoid OTC drugs unless discussed with primary care giver.

Follow-up Care

1. Stress the importance to family and client of follow-up care with their health care provider.

ESOPHAGITIS

Esophagitis is inflammation of the esophagus.

Etiology/Pathology

A common cause of esophagitis is backflow of gastric acids into the esophagus, (GERD) which causes inflamed and irritated tissue. The backflow of gastric contents can also occur with hernias, surgery, and excessive vomiting. Often gastroesophageal reflux is the direct result of a weakened lower esophageal sphincter (LES). Another common cause is infection, which may be present in immunocompromised clients, persons with bacterial, fungus, and yeast infections (Candida), viruses such as CMV (cytomegalovirus), and herpes. Oral Candida is more common in the older adult. Persons with diabetes or blood dyscrasias (leukemia) are also at higher risk for esophagitis. The client experiences dysphagia, achalasia, oral lesions or thrush, odynophagia, and anorexia resulting in significant weight loss.

General Nursing Care

1. Provide for comfort measures through pain management.
2. Maintain a supportive environment.
3. Include client in developing plan of care.

Nursing Diagnoses

1. Pain related to esophageal spasms secondary to infections.
2. Altered body image related to weight loss.

3. High risk for injury due to aspiration related to backflow of gastric juices.

Interventions, Treatments, Alternative Treatments

1. Administer pain medication as needed.
2. Teach client to avoid spicy, fatty, grilled, and smoked foods.
3. Teach client to drink warm fluids, no caffeine or carbonated drinks.
4. Administer or prepare to administer antifungal medications such as ketoconazole and fluconazole. If these antifungal medications are ineffective, prepare to administer or administer Amphotericin B.
5. Teach client about tests that may be performed esophagogastroduodenoscopy (EGD) with or without a biopsy, upper GI and small bowel series, endoscopy, throat culture, and brushing of the esophagus for a culture.
6. Teach the client the importance of fastidious oral hygiene at least three times a day.

Health Promotion and Quality of Life Issues

1. Teach client about effects of alcohol, smoking, and drug use.
2. Support client in making own decisions on what their expectations are on quality of life issues.
3. Inform client of the importance of adhering to plan of care and that failure to do so could result in Barrett's esophagus, (normal squamous cell epithelium in lower esophagus is replaced by columnar epithelium, which is more resistant to the gastric acids (pepsin & gastrin) which protect the lining of the esophagus. However, this new epithelium is precancerous and can lead to cancer of the esophagus.

Home Management and Self-Care Issues

1. Teach client and significant others to notify primary care-giver if symptoms are exacerbated.
2. Consult with primary caregiver before administering OTC drugs or alternative treatments.

3. Teach client to keep head of bed elevated 8–12 inches or lie on left side to prevent gastric acid reflux.

Follow-up Care

1. Stress the importance to family and client of follow-up care with their health care provider.

REFERENCES

CHID Digestive Diseases (1999). *Hiatal hernia: Understanding a common problem*. Retrieved August 17, 2002, from *http://www.chid.nih.gov/netacgi/nph*.

Ignaatavius, D., & Workman, L. (Eds.) (2002). *Medical surgical nursing: Critical thinking for collaborative care*. Philadelphia: W. B. Sanders.

Lyder, C. (1998). Gastrointestinal disorders. In A. Luggen, S. Travis, & S. Meiner (Eds.), *NGNA Core Curriculum for Gerontological Advanced Practice Nurses* (pp. 521–525). Thousand Oaks: SAGE Publications, Ltd.1

Mayo Clinic (February 2002). *Trouble Swallowing*. Retrieved August 17, 2002 from *http//www.mayoclinic.com*.

National Guideline Clearinghouse (1999, July). *American Gastroenterological Association medical position statement on treatment of patients with dysphagia caused by benign disorders of the distal esophagus*. Retrieved August 17, 2002, from *http/www.guide line.gov/VIEWS/summary.asp*

—3—

Gastroesophageal Reflux Disease

Catherine Hill

Once a month, more than 40% of U.S. citizens experience symptoms of gastroesophageal reflux disease (GERD) (Bilhartz & Croft, 2000). But only a small number of symptomatic patients seek medical advice for their symptoms. Although the last few years have produced more geriatric specific research on this problem, we still lack large-scale, rigorous scientific research on which to base our clinical practice. Current medical geriatric research on GERD, while limited, is more abundant than nursing research. However, it is focused primarily on geriatric surgical outcomes after laparoscopic fundoplication (Nissen antireflux surgery). Current nursing research focuses on patient responses to traditional interventions in the adult population without consideration of the emerging paradigm on pathophysiology.

So, necessarily and appropriately for this discussion of geriatric considerations on the nature and management of GERD, we begin with the current medical literature. In essence, today's medical and nursing approaches to geriatric GERD are based on yesterday's disproven theories. Rationales for some medical treatment and related nursing interventions associated with this geriatric medical diagnosis, therefore, will lack some substance. Always focused on the geriatric patient, age-specific risks, and the human response to disease, today's nursing approach needs to be based on nursing theory. Orem's Self-Care Deficit Theory of Nursing supports a comprehensive assessment of the geriatric GERD patient, valid data for nursing diagnosis development, and relevant problems for nursing intervention, following an explanation of the current medical literature on disease definition, etiology, and pathology.

DEFINITIONS

The current definition of GERD has remained rather nonspecific. However, the current understanding of its etiology and pathology contains some very specific surprises. Current research has cast significant doubt on the supposed mechanisms of GERD development, leaving the current treatment recommendations scientifically unsupported. This period of transition into a greater understanding of the basic anatomical and physiological underpinnings of this disorder in adults will no doubt yield new clinical treatment approaches. While gastroesophageal reflux (GER) is the simple retrograde movement of gastric contents back into the esophagus, it poses significant diagnostic challenges in the elderly. Often these patients do not report the classic symptoms of younger adults (Ramirez, 2000). Frequently the symptoms of water brash, sour mouth, indigestion, regurgitation, and heartburn (pyrosis) are the terms used to describe typical adult GER symptoms (Bilhartz & Croft, 2000). These classic symptoms usually warn of pathological function before the occurrence of esophageal ulceration and bleeding (Ramirez, 2000). This lack of classic presentation in the elderly makes understanding the definition, etiology, and pathology of the disorder crucial to effective nursing care.

GERD is defined as "any symptoms or histopathological changes that result from reflux of gastric contents into the esophagus" (Bilhartz & Croft, 2000, p. 2). Experienced by 4 out of 10 Americans in the last month, GERD is virtually ubiquitous in all settings. Heartburn and regurgitation are hallmarks of GERD found in 70% of older adults (Bilhartz & Croft, 2000). Often described as retrosternal burning which moves from the stomach into the throat, heartburn has been found by pH monitoring to be the cause in 20% to 50% of noncardiac chest pain cases (Bilhartz & Croft, 2000). Water brash is an unfamiliar term to some providers and refers to the sudden appearance of sour, salty fluid in the mouth. Table 3.1 lists the typical and atypical adult symptoms. Two-thirds to three-fourths of adult GERD patients are mildly obese smokers who complain of postprandial, retrosternal burning that is worse after large meals containing alcohol, chocolate, or fatty and/or spicy food. Symptoms are generally

TABLE 3.1   Categories of GERD Symptoms

Typical Symptoms	Atypical Symptoms
Heartburn	Chest pain
Regurgitation	Cough
Dysphagia	Wheezing
Odonophagia	Dyspnea
Water brash	Hoarseness
Belching	Throat clearing
	Globus sensation
	Halitosis

worse with recumbency or bending over, and are improved by antacids according to Bilhartz and Croft (2000). Traditionally, adults seek medical treatment due to the classic symptoms of odonophagia and burning chest pain (Ramirez, 2000). Unfortunately, this common symptom-based approach to identification and treatment of GERD overlooks the fact that the elderly typically experience "regurgitation, dysphagia, dyspepsia, vomiting, and noncardiac chest pain" or no symptoms at all (Ramirez, 2000, p. 756). Since symptoms are an important part of today's working definition of GERD, the existing symptom-based definition and classic adult patient presentation is less helpful and potentially harmful, in identifying geriatric GERD cases.

ETIOLOGY

Reflux is common in normal people as well as those with GERD (Katzka, Delaney, Forman, & Moayyedi, 2000). Normally, the tonically contracted lower esophageal sphincter (LES) and crural diaphragm serve as anatomical and functional barriers that prevent gastric contents from refluxing into the esophagus. The normal resting pressure of the 3 to 4 cm long LES is 10 to 30 mm Hg higher than the stomach. LES pressure decreases after meals but increases with a supine position. The crural diaphragm helps prevent reflux by increasing resistance during inspiration and at time of increased intra-abdominal pressure (Bilhartz & Croft, 2000). The mucous neck cells, pyloric glands, peptic cells, and parietal cells of the stomach normally secrete thirty percent of their response to a meal at the time of anticipation or the odor of food. Sixty percent of the acid response occurs with distention of the stomach and the final ten percent occurs with distention of the small bowel. The pancreas contributes to neutralization of stomach acids by secreting bicarbonate ions and water into the duodenum (Guyton & Hall, 2001). All of these mechanisms should be considered in assessing and planning the care of a potential geriatric GERD patient.

Once believed to be the result of a hypotensive LES, GERD is now recognized as being multifactorial since fewer than one fourth of reflux episodes are associated with low LES pressures by manometric testing on patients (Bilhartz & Croft, 2000). While limited geriatric-specific etiology research exists, most GERD patients have normal LES pressures, but experience brief, transient relaxation that correlates poorly with esophageal damage. Even the role of caustic refluxate is also now believed to be of limited importance except in special situations (Katzka, 2000). This brings the widespread use of empiric pharmacological treatment into question. In geriatric patients, abnormal salivation can exacerbate GERD (Luette et al., 1993) and may contribute to an increased incidence in the elderly. Along with the loss of taste sensation, the salivary glands lose efficiency as we age. Controlled by the parasympathetic nervous system, during adulthood, the salivary glands produce copious quantities of a watery mucous secretion containing a high concentration of bicarbonate ions (Guyton & Hall, 2001). Residual refluxed acid is partially neutralized by saliva; if salivation is abnormally depressed, the neutralizing capacity of saliva will be lost. The elderly are at particular risk for decreased salivation related to sympathetic nervous system activation during stress, decreased hydration, natural aging changes, and increased medication use. Research has shown that cigarette smokers and patients using anticholinergic medications have significantly reduced salivation (Kahrilas & Gupta, 1989). Several drugs and foods decrease LES pressure and may increase a patient's risk for reflux. While studies have not proven causation, the items in Table 3.2 have been linked to worsening of reflux symptoms and their avoidance forms a part of the management of geriatric GERD patients.

PATHOLOGY

GERD develops histologically when the normal protective mechanisms of the esophagus fail. Histological changes, symptoms, and risk of complication occur as the esophagus is injured and the reparative process fails. Considering the majority of symptomatic adults do not seek medical treatment, it is easy to infer that many reach old age with years of exposure

TABLE 3.2 Foods and Drugs Known to Affect Esophageal Tone

Substances	Increase LES tone	Decrease LES tone
Drugs	Alpha-agonists	Alpha-antagonists
	Beta-blockers	Beta-agonists
	Cholinergics	Anticholinergics
	Antacids	Theophylline
	Metoclopramide	Somatostatin
	Cisapride	Calcium Channel Blockers
		Dopamine
		Diazepam
		Progesterone
		Morphine
Foods	Protein	Fat
		Chocolate
		Onion
		Peppermint
		Ethanol

to the mechanisms of disease. According to Castell in his book *Gastroesophageal Reflux Disease* (1985), little correlation exists between the severity of symptoms and severity of pathology. This is also noted in Bilhartz and Croft's *Gastrointestinal Disease in Primary Care* (2000) yet the treatment recommendations include pharmacological therapy for symptoms that fail to respond to lifestyle modifications.

Since they are known to report less severe, different, or no symptoms (Richter, 2000) the prolonged exposure to acid over the years makes the elderly more likely to experience esophagitis, peptic strictures, and Barrett's esophagus. This may explain the widespread use of pharmacological therapy by medical professionals. Since empiric therapy for the symptomatic GERD patient is routine (Wilcox, Heudebert, Klapow, Shewchuck, & Casebeer, 2001), our elderly who sought out treatment as adults may avoid serious complications. A recent 24-hour esophageal pH monitoring study performed in China on 20 healthy elderly without GERD symptoms was compared with 69 suspected elderly GERD subjects (Wu, Wang, & Li, 1999). The results revealed that 51.6% of elderly patients with GERD symptoms did not have endoscopic evidence of esophagitis. With the relative lack of age specific research, the elderly GERD patient's need for ongoing care and symptom management is a significant challenge.

GENERAL NURSING CARE

Gastroesophageal reflux disease is a chronic recurring disorder, which is widespread, especially in Western societies (Shridhar, Huang, O'Brien, & Hunt, 1996). The most common reason for the use of over-the-counter antacids is postprandial reflux, most often while in the upright position (Bilhartz & Croft, 2000). Since the definition of GERD depends heavily on patient reported symptoms, the elderly are logically undertreated and at increased risk for poor outcomes. The nursing process provides an excellent framework for the general nursing care of the geriatric GERD patient, as well as the patient who may have not been formally "diagnosed" yet. A comprehensive assessment is required, because a focused assessment will be less than adequate and possibly harmful when dealing with a multifactorial disease such as GERD. Figure 3.1 shows a theory-based comprehensive assessment tool for the first phase of the nursing process. History taking should utilize appropriate age-related techniques (Fig. 3.2).

The geriatric history is very important in establishing the nursing approach to GERD. Specific attention to the following aspects will ensure appropriate nursing diagnosis and interventions: (1) weight loss, (2) use of supplemental feedings, (3) 24-hour diet recall, (4) frequency/size of feedings, (5) food preferences, (6) the patient's evaluation of smell and taste, (7) social isolation when eating, (8) daily vitamin/mineral use, (9) correct fitting dentures, (10) broken teeth or cavities, (11) mouth care routines, (12) dry mouth or eyes, (13) fluid intake, (14) use of stool softeners or laxatives, (15) daily activity/endurance, (16) access to/safety of food, (17) cooking facilities, (18) use of over-the-counter medicines, (19) ability to sleep flat, (20) night awakenings, and (21) poor wound healing. When evaluating a geriatric GERD patient it is important to identify whether over-the-counter H2 blockers (cimetidine, ranitidine) are in use. In undiagnosed elderly patients the routine use of over-the-counter H2 blockers, and the presence of hoarseness, cough, or dyspnea indicate the need for medical evaluation. Assess the duration of self-treatment, amount of medication, frequency of H2 blocker use, and existence of breakthrough symptoms or weight loss to decide the urgency of your referral.

Physical assessment of the geriatric GERD patient is generally normal (Bilhartz & Croft, 2000). However, it can be helpful to exclude other problems to establish a baseline and include an examination of general appearance, height, weight, body mass index, facial symmetry, oral cavity, swallowing, mucous membranes, skin condition, chest, abdomen, reflexes, bone deformities, and strength and range of motion.

1. Client Profile
    a. Personal characteristics
        1) Name
        2) Age
        3) Sex
        4) Marital status
        5) Ethnic orientation
        6) Religious orientation
        7) Educational level
        8) Language
        9) Occupational history (type of job, duration)
        10) Interest, hobbies, recreational activities
    b. Current health orientation
        1) What do you consider to be healthy about you?
        2) What are your health goals?
    c. Family characteristics
        1) Family members/significant others (age, relationship to client)
        2) Type of family form
        3) Family structure
            a) Role structure
            b) Value systems
            c) Communication pattern
            d) Power structure
        4) Family function
            a) Affective function
            b) Socialization and social placement function
            c) Reproductive function
            d) Family coping function
            e) Economic function
            f) Provision of physical necessities
    d. Environmental characteristics
        1) Physical setting: home (characteristics, safety hazards, spatial adequacy, provision of privacy)
        2) Physical setting: neighborhood and community, including geographic mobility patterns; presence of environmental hazards
        3) Associations and transactions of the family with the community, and perception and feelings about neighborhood and community; include accessibility of health-care facilities, human services
2. Universal Self-Care Requisites
    a. Air
        1) Health habits

FIGURE 3.1   Patient history based on Dorothea E. Orem's self-care deficit theory of nursing (Dennis, 1997).

        a)   Hygiene (bathing and grooming practices, oral hygiene, feminine hygiene, special cultural practices)

        b)   Patterns of oxygenation (special aids)

    2)   Review of systems

        a)   Skin: rashes, pruritis, scaling, lesions, turgor, skin growths, tumors, masses, pigmentation changes, or discoloration

        b)   Hair: changes in amount, texture, character; alopecia, use of dyes

        c)   Nails: changes in appearance, texture, capillary refill

        d)   Breast: pain, skin changes, lesions, dimpling, lumps, nipple discharge, mastectomy.

        e)   Respiratory system: nose (pain or trauma, olfaction, sensitivity, epistaxis, discharge); shortness of breath, dyspnea, chronic cough, sputum production, hemoptysis; history of asthma, wheezing, or noise with breathing

        f)   Cardiovascular system: palpitations, heart murmur, varicose veins, history of heart disease; hypertension, chest pains, orthopnea

        g)   Peripheral vascular system: coldness, numbness, discoloration, peripheral edema, intermittent claudication

b.   Water

    1)   Health habits

        a)   Patterns of fluid intake

        b)   Fluid likes/dislikes

        c)   Fluid temperature preferences

    2)   Review of systems

        a)   Hydration: dehydration, excessive dryness, sweating; odors, edema, polydipsia

        b)   Parenteral fluids (IV blood administration, hyperalimentation)

c.   Food

    1)   Health habits

        a)   24-hour diet recall: frequency of meals, quantities

        b)   Foods likes and dislikes

        c)   Dietary modifications (cultural, religious, medical)

        d)   Food preparation

        e)   Meal environment

        f)   Food budgeting

        g)   Food supplements (vitamins, minerals, fluorinated water supply)

        h)   Weight gain/loss patterns

        i)   Problems related to ingestion/digestion (special aids)

        j)   Related prescribed or patent medicines

FIGURE 3.1 *(continued)*

Gastroesophageal Reflux Disease

31

2) Review of systems
 a) Mouth: teeth, gums, tongue, buccae, chewing difficulty
 b) Throat: pain, lesions, dysarthria, dysphagia, history of strep infections
 c) Gastrointestinal system: pain, nausea/vomiting, acid indigestion, ulcer history, polyphagia, present height-weight status
d. Elimination
 1) Health habits
  a) Daily patterns (bladder, bowel)
  b) Aids (fluids, foods, medications, enemas)
 2) Review of systems
  a) Bladder: polyuria, oliguria, dysuria, nocturia, incontinence, difficulty stopping or starting stream, force of stream, dribbling, pain or burning on urination, urinary tract infections
  b) Bowel: pain, diarrhea, constipation (acute or chronic), flatulence, hemorrhoids, stool characteristics (color, consistency, amount)
  c) Surgical opening: draining wounds, ostomies
  d) Genitalia: perineal rashes and irritations, lesions, unusual discharge (amount, color, consistency)
e. Activity and rest
 1) Health habits
  a) Activity patterns: means of ambulation (safety concerns, aids); level of activity (home, work, leisure); regular exercise program
  b) Sleep/rest patterns: circadian rhythms; time and duration of sleep; use of supportive aids (sedatives, alcohol, pillows), devices (reading, music)
 2) Review of systems
  a) Musculoskeletal system: muscle strength/weakness, muscle tone, range of motion, pain, fatigue, swelling, stiffness, contractures
  b) Neurological system: numbness, tingling; discrimination between heat, cold, and touch; unusual movements (tremors, seizures); paralysis; dizziness, headache, loss of consciousness, memory changes; intolerance to heat and cold
f. Solitude and social interaction
 1) Health habits
  a) Communication
  b) Social interactions
  c) Sexuality: attitudes toward own sexuality (femininity/masculinity), sexual orientation, frequency of sexual activity, satisfaction with sexual activity, contraceptive measures
  d) Solitude: opportunities and selected activities during solitude

FIGURE 3.1 (continued)

2)   Review of systems
    a)   Ear: pain, discharge, tinnitus, decrease/increase in hearing, use of hearing aids
    b)   Eye: pain, discharge, vision, corrective lenses, blurred vision, diplopia, night blindness, color vision
    c)   Reproductive system

g.   Hazards to human life, human functioning, and human well-being
    1)   Personal safety practices
    2)   Social habits (drugs, alcohol, tobacco, coffee-tea-cola; specify level of use)

h.   Normalcy: promotion of human functioning and development within social groups in accord with human potential, known limitations, and the human desire to be normal
    1)   Health habits
        a)   Health resources used (medical, dental, vision and hearing, screening programs, immunizations, counseling)
        b)   Personal health practices (stress/anxiety management, meditation, relaxation techniques; self-breast exam, testicular exam)
    2)   Self concept/image
        a)   Body image (appearance, boundaries, limits, inner structure)
        b)   Mental health
            i.   Attitude
            ii.   Affect/mood
            iii. Thought processes (logical, coherent, perceptual)
            iv.   Sensorium and reasoning (levels of consciousness, orientation, memory, calculation, abstract thinking, judgment/insight, intelligence
            v.   Locus of control
            vi.   Potential for danger (harm to self/other)
        c)   Spirituality

3.   **Developmental Self-Care Requisites**
    a.   Life-cycle stage and related concerns (neonatal, infancy, toddler, preschool, school age, adolescence, early adulthood, middle adulthood, childbearing, late adulthood
    b.   Psychosexual stage (Freud)
    c.   Psychosocial stage (Erikson)
    d.   Intellectual stage (Piaget)
    e.   Moral stage (Kohlberg)
    f.   Conditions that promote or prevent normal development (life events, poor health, education)

4.   **Health Deviation Self-Care Requisites**
    a.   Present deviation
    1)   Perception of deviation
        a)   Reason for contact

FIGURE 3.1 *(continued)*

      b)   Understanding of this current alteration in health status
      c)   Feelings about present health status
      d)   Specific concerns
   2) Coping mechanisms
      a)   Past use of coping mechanisms to deal with similar alterations
      b)   Current repertoire of coping mechanisms and their adequacy
      c)   Concurrent stresses (life events)
   3) Effects of deviation on life styles
      a)   Psychological
      b)   Physiological
      c)   Financial
 b. Past history of health deviations
   1) Adult illness
   2) Childhood illness
   3) Accidents/injuries
   4) Hospitalizations
   5) Allergies
      a)   Drugs
      b)   Food
      c)   Other
   6) Medications
      a)   Prescription
      b)   Self-prescribed
 c. Family health history
   1) Relatives living or dead with similar health deviations
   2) Presence of any hereditary diseases (diabetes, hypertension, heart disease)

FIGURE 3.1 *(continued)*

NURSING DIAGNOSIS AND PLAN OF CARE

Approach the geriatric GERD patient armed with a comprehensive history and focused physical assessment. Some patient problems should be apparent from the assessment phase based on your knowledge of medical therapies and human response to illness. Using the completed Figure 3.1 assessment, make a list of patient problems, then select potentially suitable North American Nursing Diagnosis Association (NANDA) (2002) diagnoses from Table 3.3. Confirm that your patient meets the "defining characteristics" of each nursing diagnosis by using the assessment information. Make notes on the assessment form of additional information or assessments you may need to make after reviewing the "defining characteristics" (Carpenito, 2002). Each nursing diagnosis should use a three-part format—identify

- Pace interview according to client's energy level
- Sit close if hearing or visual impairment; encourage the use of glasses or hearing aid
- Speak and respond at a pace the client can comprehend; clearly enunciate words
- Use words and language appropriate for the client's age and level of understanding
- Repeat questions if necessary; allow time to respond
- Give prompting on answers and explain exactly what you need to know
- Use reminiscing strategies and association strategies to help patients
- Watch for evidence of fatigue; be prepared to collect information in multiple encounters
- Avoid ageism or demeaning comments
- Use a conversational style asking one question at a time
- Obtain additional information from family or friends if possible
- Frequently there are multiple comorbidities and medications
- Use reality testing, close proximity, and good eye contact in confused or disoriented clients

FIGURE 3.2   Geriatric interview techniques.

the problem, its etiology, and symptoms (Carpenito, 2002). Table 3.3 organizes a selection of common geriatric GERD-related NANDA diagnoses according to the categories of treatment-related, pathophysiologic, maturational, personal, environmental, potential complications, and collaborative problems. Considering the multifactorial influences on GERD, nursing's holistic approach, and the complex history of the geriatric patient, an accurate and thorough diagnosis is challenging and critical to your success. Look specifically for "geriatric considerations" listed with each nursing diagnosis. Since these are too numerous to list here, refer to *Nursing Diagnosis: Application to Clinical Practice* by Carpenito (2002). Table 3.3 will assist you in addressing six of the seven categories related to geriatric GERD. Only the wellness category has been omitted due to the disease focus of this chapter.

INTERVENTIONS, TREATMENTS, ALTERNATIVE THERAPY

Given that geriatric issues involve atypical symptoms such as altered pharmacokinetics, polypharmacy, drug interactions, and an increased risk of complications in the elderly, effective nursing management of older patients with GERD can be a challenge. Typically, treatment for the geriatric patient

TABLE 3.3 Nursing Diagnoses to Consider for Geriatric GERD Patient

Treatment-related	Pathophysiologic	Maturational	Personal/Environmental	Potential Complications	Collaborative Problems
Nausea	Deficient fluid volume	Activity intolerance related to aging or impaired physical mobility	Ineffective coping	Risk for aspiration	Negative nitrogen balance
Effective or Ineffective Therapeutic Management	Disturbed sleep pattern	Impaired adjustment	Deficient knowledge	Imbalanced nutrition: less than body requirements	Fluid or electrolyte imbalances
Constipation related to antacids	Adult failure to thrive	Anxiety related to threat to self-concept	Ineffective health maintenance	Impaired oral mucous membranes	Alcohol or tobacco withdrawal
Diarrhea related to medication treatment	Fatigue	Ineffective thermoregulation	Noncompliance	Impaired tissue integrity	Proton pump inhibitor therapy adverse effects
Health-Seeking Behaviors	Nausea	Impaired communication related to hearing impairment	Self-care deficit: feeding Instrumental self-care deficit	Risk for imbalanced body temperature	H2 blocker therapy adverse effects

(continued)

TABLE 3.3 *(continued)*

Treatment-related	Pathophysiologic	Maturational	Personal/ Environmental	Potential Complications	Collaborative Problems
Fear related to laparoscopic fundoplication procedure, diagnostic tests	Acute or chronic pain	Readiness for enhanced community coping related to community programs	Disabled family coping	Hopelessness Powerlessness	Prokinetic therapy adverse effects
Acute pain related to laparoscopic fundoplication incision, flatus, immobility		Disturbed sensory perception	Ineffective community coping related to knowledge of resources	Risk for infection	GI bleeding
		Impaired urinary elimination	Deficient diversional activity	Risk for injury	Esophageal perforation
			Impaired home maintenance	Risk for loneliness	Barrett's esophagus

follows three stages or phases in a cumulative fashion. Rarely will a patient have an infectious, trauma tic, or iatrogenic cause for their symptoms. Occasionally, the patient or family has a history of gastric cancer or previous gastrointestinal disease. These two previously mentioned circumstances would necessitate immediate referral for medical evaluation. However, for most patients, lifestyle modifications and acid neutralization provide the initial therapy. Often, stage-one therapies are instituted by patients who do not seek medical care. Through trial and error many patients discover and avoid foods or medicines that worsen their symptoms, use over-the-counter antacids or H2 blockers and avoid lying down after meals. As the nurse becomes involved, stage-one therapy includes education in addition to comprehensive lifestyle modification and acid neutralization with antacids or alginates (Table 3.4). Typically, twenty percent of symptomatic GERD patients can be managed by this conservative approach if reflux esophagitis does not exist. Historically, most symptomatic patients require aggressive therapy for initial treatment and maintenance. Stage-one patients who experience breakthrough symptoms or symptoms that last more than two to four weeks warrant medical evaluation.

Stage-two therapy for GERD is implemented when the patient sees a nurse practitioner or physician. Often stage two begins with reinforcement of lifestyle modifications and education after a comprehensive history and physical. In spite of the lack of clear scientific evidence on hyperacidity in the pathogenesis of GERD, in most cases an empiric trial of acid suppression occurs (Bilhartz & Croft, 2000). If successful, in symptom management, the medication continues under medical supervision. Table 3.5 outlines the typical progression of pharmacological management options (Bilhartz & Croft, 2000).

Stage-three GERD therapy involves surgical intervention. No consensus currently exists about who should be offered surgery. However, some guidelines have been offered by Bilhartz and Croft (2000) as listed in Table 3.6. Several recent studies have explored the efficacy of laparoscopic antireflux surgery in the elderly (Khajanchee, Urbach, Butler, Hansen, & Swanstrom, 2002; Granderath, Kamolz, Schweiger, Bammer, & Pointer, 2001; Kamolz, Bammer, Granderath, Pasiut, & Pointer, 2001) due to the perceived higher surgical complication rate and high cost of pharmacological management of geriatric GERD. Three out of four of the recent studies found improved acid reflux symptoms without significant surgical complications for geriatric GERD patients. Only Terry and colleagues (2001) noted three deaths, all of which involved elderly patients, out of 1000 patients who underwent laparoscopic fundoplications for GERD and whose

TABLE 3.4   Stage-One Treatment of GERD

Category	Interventions/Rationales
Body Position	Elevate the head of the bed 2 to 6 inches Do not use pillows because the patient slides down at night Rationale: upright position decreases frequency of reflux
Postprandial Recumbency	Do not lie down for at least 2 hours after meals Rationale: Gravity helps stomach emptying and decreases stomach distention
Dietary Modifications	Avoid the following foods: Fat Tomatoes Chocolate Citric acids Ethanol Cola Coffee Onions Carminatives Tea Rationale: decrease LES tone by increasing acid which irritates mucosa
Smoking Cessation	Stop or decrease smoking Rationale: decreases LES tone and increases frequency of reflux
Weight Loss	Lose weight if you are obese Rationale: increased abdominal fat increases abdominal pressure, increasing reflux
Meal Size Reduction	Small frequent meals Rationale: avoids gastric distention
Antacids and Alginates	Take antacids at bedtime and one to three hours after each meal The combination of antacid and alginate is more effective than either alone Rationale: reduces acidity

TABLE 3.5 Stage-Two Pharmacologic Therapy for GERD

Medication	Actions
Histamine Receptor Blockers	Provides a reversible histamine blockade of the parietal cells Commonly cimetidine, ranitidine, nizatidine, famotidine Reduces acid 60% to 70% Heals esophagitis in 8 weeks in 28% to 66% of patients
Proton Pump Inhibitors	Provides an irreversible inhibition of the parietal cells Reduces acid production by 95% Heals esophagitis in 8 weeks in 74% to 88% of patients
Prokinetic Agents	Increases LES resting tone Commonly bethanechol, metoclopramide

TABLE 3.6 Guidelines for Antireflux Surgery

Recommended	Not Recommended
Patient preference in the young and otherwise healthy	Unidentified etiology of symptoms
Refractory complications including asthma and laryngitis	Esophageal dysmotility
Esophageal bleeding or perforation	Patients with substantial co-morbidities
Failure to heal with prolonged proton pump inhibitor therapy	
Defective lower esophageal sphincter	

mean age was 49. With increased geriatric-specific research we may soon have more evidenced-based recommendations for the elderly.

Alternative, natural, or complementary medicine views digestive health as central to long-term good health and identifies heartburn, gaseousness, abdominal fullness, and indigestion as common presenting patient complaints (Pizzorno & Murray, 1999). The medical diagnosis of GERD corresponds to the naturopathic diagnosis of maldigestion (Pizzorno & Murray, 1999). Empiric treatment with antacids, H2 blockers, and other medications is contraindicated due to their belief that this approach treats symptoms without identification of the cause of the symptoms. Naturopathic health care providers cite the reduction of gastric acidity, by raising the pH to 3.5 with medications as a harmful practice which impairs protein digestion and mineral disassociation while relieving stomach irritation. In addition, they believe the pH change adversely effects gastrointestinal flora promoting an overgrowth of Helicobacter pylori (Pizzorno & Murray, 1999). Many natural medicine providers believe the common symptoms of GERD can easily be attributable to many other digestive problems. Problem identification through differential diagnosis is routine before advising treatment. Usually, the diagnosis is confirmed by a "comprehensive digestive stool analysis" (CDSA), which is a diagnostic tool for the analysis of digestion, the colonic environment, and absorption. Table 3.7 outlines the components of CDSA testing including individual tests, the corresponding digestive function evaluated, and the disease states that may be involved. Using history and physical techniques similar to allopathic medicine, the practitioner of alternative or natural medicine will establish one of the diagnoses listed in Table 3.7 and institute treatment. Nursing interventions based on this paradigm are beyond the scope of this chapter.

HEALTH PROMOTION AND QUALITY OF LIFE ISSUES

While there is little correlation between the severity of symptoms and the severity of pathology, symptomatic patients have a significantly reduced quality of life. Most geriatric GERD patients with daily symptoms do not have esophagitis on endoscopy but still require daily medication for symptom control (Glise, 1995). Symptom duration in patients seeking treatment is often greater than 5 years. Unfortunately, after treatment, relapse is seen in a majority of cases. Symptoms of reflux and dyspepsia affect several aspects of daily life; consequently, quality of life is lower in GERD patients (Glise, 1995). Various quality of life assessment tools have been developed over the years, however none specifically for the geriatric GERD patient. Spitzer and Dobson (1981) developed a concise, easy to use quality of life instrument for use on cancer patients that has been successfully used in other chronic illnesses (Fig. 3.3). The quality of life index they developed is derived from the patient's evaluation of the categories: activity, daily living, health, support, and outlook. With a maximum score of ten and a minimum score of zero, through serial monitoring spaced two or more weeks apart, the patient's quality of life trends offer helpful

TABLE 3.7 Natural Medicine Approach to GERD: CDSA Testing

Function Tested Disease States	Component Analyzed	Potential Diagnosis
Digestion	Triglycerides	Pancreatic insufficiency
	Chymotrypsin	Pancreatic insufficiency
		Hypoacidity
		Cystic fibrosis
	Iso-butyrate, iso-valerate, n-valerate	Pancreatic insufficiency
		Malabsorption
		Bacterial fermentation
		Maldigestion
	Meat & vegetable fibers	Hypoacidity
		Pancreatic insufficiency
Absorption	Total fecal fat	Maldigestion
		Malabsorption
	Long chain fatty acids	Gastric mucosal disease
		Pancreatic insufficiency
	Cholesterol	Mucosal malabsorption
		Mucosal epithelial cell breakdown
	Total short chain fatty acids	Abnormal colonic flora
		Insufficient dietary fiber
Microbiology	Lactobacilli	Abnormal colonic flora
	Bifidobacteria	Abnormal colonic flora
	E. coli	Abnormal colonic flora
	C. albicans	Abnormal colonic flora
	C. tropicalis	Abnormal colonic flora
	Rhodotorula	Abnormal colonic flora
	Geotrichum	Abnormal colonic flora
Metabolic Markers	n-Butyrate	Colon cancer
		Ulcerative colitis
		Inflammatory bowel
	Beta-glucuronidase	Increased cancer risk
		Dietary insufficiency
		Abnormal colonic flora
	PH	Inadequate dietary fiber
	Short chain fatty acid distribution	Abnormal colonic flora
		Bacterial infection
		Colon cancer

(continued)

TABLE 3.7   *(continued)*

Function Tested Disease States	Component Analyzed	Potential Diagnosis
Immunology	Fecal sigA	Abnormal colonic flora Infection Allergy
Macroscopic Observations	Color	Diarrhea Abnormal colonic flora GI bleeding Bile duct blockage Pancreatic insufficiency
	Mucous	Irritable bowel syndrome Inflammation Diverticulitis Abscess
	Pus	Irritable bowel syndrome Inflammation Diverticulitis Abscess
	Occult blood	Hemorrhoids Too much red meat Colon cancer
Dysbiosis Index	Metabolic and microbiologic factors: calculated	May support any of the above

general information on the success of the medical therapeutics and nursing care plan.

HOME MANAGEMENT AND SELF-CARE ISSUES

As discussed in the interventions, treatments, and alternative therapy section, often the initial stage-one therapy is implemented by the patient before seeking medical treatment (Table 3.4). Many excellent patient teaching tools and handouts exist for GERD, however none are specific to the elderly. The geriatric considerations mentioned by Carpenito (2002) are probably most helpful in developing an individualized home care plan.

Overview: A simple instrument developed to allow rapid assessment of a patient's quality of life. It was developed for patients with cancer but can be used in other clinical situations.

Scoring

- the finding for each parameter that most closely matches the patient's current condition is selected and the corresponding points assigned
- typically the patient is assessed at intervals of weeks to months

Parameter	Finding	Points
activity	working or studying full time or nearly so in usual occupation or managing own household or participating in voluntary activities	2
	working or studying in usual occupation or managing own household or participating in voluntary activities but requiring major assistance or reduction in hours worked in a sheltered situation or on sick leave	1
	not working or studying in any capacity and not managing own household	0
Daily living	able to eat, wash, toilet, and dress self; able to use public transport or drive own car	2
	requires assistance with daily activities and transport but able to perform light tasks	1
	unable to manage personal care or light tasks and/or unable to leave own home or institution	0
health	appearing to feel well or reporting feeling "great" most of the time	2
	lacking in energy or not feeling entirely "up to par" more than occasionally	1
	feeling very ill or "lousy," weak, and washed out most of the time or patient unconscious	0
support	having good relationships with others and receiving strong support from at least one family member or friend	2
	receiving limited support from family or friends because of conditions	1
	receiving support from family/friends infrequently or only when absolutely necessary or patient unconscious	0
outlook	usually appeared calm and positive in outlook, accepting, and in control of personal circumstances and surroundings	2
	troubled sometimes because not fully in control of personal circumstances or has been having periods of anxiety or depression	1
	seriously confused or very frightened, or consistently anxious or depressed, or patient unconscious	0

FIGURE 3.3 Quality of life assessment.

QL index =

QL = (points for activity) + (points for daily living) + (points for health) + (points for support) + (points for outlook)

Interpretation:

- Maximum score: 10
- Minimum score: 0
- High scores better than low scores
- Scores 0–3 are considered very low scores
- Best interpreted by trend analysis; increasing scores indicates improvement while decreasing scores deterioration

Limitations

- Because of the intervals between assessments, this is better geared for patients with chronic conditions rather than acute disease

FIGURE 3.3 *(continued)*

Selection of NANDA nursing diagnoses which meet major criteria (NANDA, 2001), utilization of three-part diagnostic statements, incorporation of Carpenito's (2002) "Geriatric Considerations," use of Nursing Interventions Classifications (NIC) (McCloskey & Bulechek, 2000) and regular re-evaluation using Nursing Outcomes Classifications (NOC) (Johnson et al., 2000) will maximize the strength of nursing management during the evolution of medical knowledge in the near future (see Table 3.3).

FOLLOW-UP CARE

GERD is often a relapsing disease. Some develop local complications such as strictures or Barrett's esophagus. Others may have extra esophageal complications. Symptomatic geriatric patients diagnosed with GERD should receive routine follow-up every one to three months (Bilhartz & Croft, 2000). Asymptomatic patients not on medication warrant annual follow-up. Patients who are dissatisfied with their current medical treatment or symptom control could consult a reputable naturopathic provider for additional testing and treatment recommendations. Complete abandonment of medical follow-up is never recommended.

REFERENCES

Bilhartz, L. E., & Croft, C. L. (2000). *Gastrointestinal disease in primary care*. Philadelphia: Lippincott Williams & Wilkins.

Carpenito, L. J. (2002). *Nursing diagnosis: Application to clinical practice*. Philadelphia: Lippincott.

Castell, D. O. (1985). *Gastroesophageal reflux disease*. New York: Futura Publishing Company.

Glise, H. (1995). Quality of life and cost of therapy in reflux disease. *Scandinavian Journal of Gastroenterology, 210*, 38–42.

Granderath, F. A., Kamolz, T., Schweiger, U. M., Bammer, T., & Pointer, R. (2001). Outcome after laparascopic antireflux surgery: Fundoplication and refundoplication in the elderly. *Der Chirurg; Zeitschrift fur alle Gebiete der operativen Medizen, 72*(9), 1026–1031.

Johnson, M., Maas, M., et al. (Eds.). (2000). *Nursing outcomes classification* (2nd ed.). St. Louis, MO: Mosby.

Kahrilas, P. J., & Gupta, R. R. (1989). The effect of cigarette smoking on salivation and esophageal clearance. *Journal of Laboratory and Clinical Medicine, 114,* 418.

Kamolz, T., Bammer, T., Granderath, F. A., Pasiut, M., & Pointer, R. (2001). Quality of life and surgical outcome after laparoscopic antireflux surgery in the elderly gastroesophageal patient. *Scandinavian Journal of Gastroenterology, 36,* 116–120.

Katzka, D., Delaney, B., Forman, D., & Moayyedi, P. (2000). Gastro-oesophageal reflux disease. *Clinical Evidence, 6,* 351–363.

Khajanchee, Y. S., Urbach, D. R., Butler, N., Hansen, P. D., & Swanstrom, L. L. (2002). Laparoscopic antireflux surgery in the elderly. *Surgical Endoscopy, 16,* 25–30.

McCloskey, J., & Bulechek, G. (Eds.) (2000). Nursing interventions classification (NIC): Iowa intervention project (3rd ed.). St. Louis, MO: Mosby.

North American Nursing Diagnosis Association (2001). Nursing diagnosis: Definitions and classification, 2001–2002. Philadelphia: NANDA.

Pizzorno, J. E., & Murray, M. T. (1999). *Textbook of natural medicine* (2nd ed.). Edinburgh: Churchill Livingstone.

Ramirez, F. C. (2000). Diagnosis and treatment of gastroesophageal reflux disease in the elderly. *Cleveland Clinic Journal of Medicine, 67*(10), 755–766.

Richter, J. E. (2000). Gastroesophageal reflux disease in the older patient: Presentation, treatment and complications. *American Journal of Gastroenterology, 95*(2), 368–373.

Spitzer, W. O., Dobson, A. J., et al. (1981). Measuring the quality of life of cancer patients. *Journal of Chronic Disability, 34,* 585–597.

Sridhar, S., Huang, J., O'Brien, B. J., & Hunt, R. H. (1996). Clinical economics review: Cost-effectiveness of treatment alternatives for gastrooesophageal reflux disease. *Alimentary Pharmacology and Therapeutics, 15*(7), 691–699.

Terry, M., Smith, C. D., Branum, G. D., Galloway, K., Waring, J. P., & Hunter, J. G. (2001). Outcomes of laparoscopic fundoplication for gastroesophageal reflux disease and paraesophageal hernia. *Surgical Endoscopy, 15*(7), 691–699.

Wilcox, C. M., Heudebert, G., Klapow, J., Shewchuck, R., & Casebeer, L. (2001). Survey of primary care physicians' approach to gastroesophageal reflux disease in elderly patients. *Journals of Gerontology, Series A, Biological Sciences and Medical Sciences, 56*(8), M514–M517.

Wu, B., Wang, M., & Li, Y. (1999). Diagnosis of gastroeshopageal reflux disease in elderly subjects using 24-hour esophageal pH monitoring. *Chinese Medical Journal, 112*(4), 333–335.

—4—

Motor Dysfunctions of the Stomach

Susan D. Kowalski

Motor dysfunctions of the stomach include conditions which present acute, recurrent, or chronic symptoms relating to stasis or rapid transit of stomach contents in the absence of any obstruction (Camilleri, 1998). Commonly recognized disorders of gastric motility include 1) delaying disorders such as gastroparesis and gastric retention, and 2) rapid disorders such as dumping syndrome and tachygastria. These motor dysfunctions can cause severe alarm and discomfort for the older adult, and may seriously interfere with normal digestion and passage of food from the stomach to the small intestine.

DEFINITIONS

Gastroparesis has been defined by Dorland's Illustrated Medical Dictionary as "paralysis of the stomach" (1994, p. 1628). Gastroparesis occurs when the stomach fails to empty normally because of decreased gastric motility. When the stomach fails to contract at its normal pace and move food into the small bowel, ingested substances remain in the stomach for a prolonged period of time. Typical symptoms of gastroparesis include nausea, vomiting, early satiety, anorexia, abdominal bloating, and abdominal discomfort (NIDDK/NIH, 1999). In older adults for whom stasis and vomiting are significant problems, there may be considerable weight loss and disturbances of mineral and vitamin stores.

Gastric retention is the term commonly used to describe an acute or chronic condition where there is delayed emptying of solid or liquid contents from the stomach into the small intestine. The terms gastric retention and gastroparesis may sometimes be used interchangeably, although gastric retention refers to holding of solids and liquids in the stomach, whereas gastroparesis refers to absent or slow muscle contractions leading to the retention of contents in the stomach (See Table 4.1).

In contrast to slow gastric motility, abnormally fast stomach emptying occurs in dumping syndrome. Dumping syndrome is the sudden massive emptying of highly acidic and hyperosmotic gastric secretions into the duodenum and jejunum (Porth, 1998). This increased stomach motility is most often associated with surgical procedures of the stomach such as gastrojejunostomy and partial gastrectomy. Symptoms include nausea, weakness, sweating, palpitation, varying degrees of syncope, often a sensation of warmth, and sometimes diarrhea, occurring after ingestion of food (Dorland's Illustrated Medical Dictionary, 1994).

Tachygastria is an abnormally fast rhythm of the stomach, in which coordination of rhythmic contractions in the stomach is lost. Food enters the small intestine in fits and starts, instead of in a smooth, controlled way. This can lead to fluctuations in blood glucose, which can aggravate impaired gastric motility and emptying (D'Arrigo, 1999).

ETIOLOGY

The major causes of gastroparesis are diabetes, postviral syndromes, surgery on the vagus nerve or stomach, medications (particularly anticholinergics

TABLE 4.1   Comparison of Signs and Symptoms of Gastric Motility Disorders

Gastroparesis	Dumping Syndrome
Nausea	Nausea
Vomiting	Weakness
Early Satiety	Diaphoresis
Anorexia	Palpitations
Abdominal Bloating	Syncope
Abdominal Discomfort	Flushing
	Diarrhea

and narcotics, which slow stomach contractions), smooth muscle disorders such as amyloidosis and scleroderma, nervous system diseases such as Parkinson's disease, and metabolic disorders such as hypothyroidism. Gastroparesis is most often a complication of Type 1 diabetes (at least 20 percent of people with Type 1 diabetes will develop gastroparesis).

Dumping syndrome and accelerated gastric emptying are most commonly caused by gastric surgical procedures such as a partial or total gastrectomy, pyloroplasty, or gastrojejunostomy (Birrer, 2002). Rapid gastric emptying results from impaired relaxation of the stomach upon ingestion of food. Postprandial intragastric pressure is relatively high and results in active propulsion of liquid foods from the stomach. A high caloric (usually carbohydrate) content of the liquid phase of the meal evokes a rapid insulin response with secondary hypoglycemia (Camilleri, 1998). See Table 4.2.

PHYSIOLOGY

A review of normal gastric motility as described by Camilleri (1998) is helpful in understanding the pathology of G.I. motor dysfunctions. Changes in the speed of stomach motility can be described as either fasting or postprandial. During the fasting period a cyclic motor phenomenon called the interdigestive migrating motor complex occurs in three phases. During Phase I the stomach moves approximately once every 60–90 minutes fol-

TABLE 4.2   Etiology of Gastric Motility Disorders

Causes of Gastroparesis	Causes of Dumping Syndrome
Diabetes	Gastric Surgical Procedures:
Postviral syndromes	Partial gastrectomy
Surgery on vagus nerve	Total gastrectomy
Medications	Pyloroplasty
(anticholinergics, narcotics)	Gastrojejunostomy
Smooth muscle disorders	
(amyloidosis, scleroderma)	
Neural disease	
(Parkinson's)	
Metabolic disorders	
(Hypothyroidism)	
Paraneoplastic syndrome	

lowed by a period of quiescence. Phase II is characterized by a period of intermittent pressure activity. The stomach is most active during Phase III when contractions occur approximately three times per minute. Following the eating of food the fasting cyclic activity is replaced by irregular, fairly frequent contractions in the stomach region. The caloric content of the meal is the major determinant of the duration and pattern of these contractions. Solids and liquids exit the stomach at different rates. The healthy stomach will empty nonnutrient liquids with a half-emptying time of 20 minutes or less. Solids are initially retained selectively within the stomach until particles are digested to a size smaller than 2 mm, at which point they are emptied in a linear fashion from the stomach. Thus, there is an initial lag period for emptying of solids, followed by a more linear, postlag gastric emptying phase. The motor function of the stomach is controlled by contraction of smooth muscle cells and their integration and modulation by enteric and extrinsic nerves. Derangement of any of these intrinsic or extrinsic control mechanisms may lead to altered gut motor function.

PATHOPHYSIOLOGY

Gastroparesis. Diseases or conditions which interfere with the intrinsic or extrinsic nervous system will impact the ability of the stomach to contract in a normal fashion, thus slowing the migrating motor complex. The enteric nervous system, which comprises approximately 100 million neurons in ganglionated plexi, is organized in intricate excitatory and inhibitory programmed circuits. Disorders of the enteric nervous system are usually the result of a degenerative, immune, or inflammatory process. Virally induced gastroparesis may be the result of cytomegalovirus or Epstein-Barr virus. Degenerative disorders may infiltrate the myenteric plexus with inflammatory cells, including eosinophils. The extrinsic neural control of the gut is subdivided into the craniosacral parasympathetic outflow and the thoracolumbar sympathetic supply. Disruption of these autonomic nerves will strongly affect G.I. motility. Extrinsic neuropathic processes include vagotomy, diabetes, amyloidosis, and a paraneoplastic syndrome usually associated with small-cell carcinoma of the lung. Extrinsic neural processes can also be affected by medications, such as alpha-adrenergic agonists and anticholinergics, which decrease or halt stomach contractions and mobility. Disturbances of smooth muscle, such as systemic sclerosis and amyloidosis, may result in significant disorders of gastric emptying. Thus, although the stomach muscle may be enervated, it is unable to respond to sensory stimuli.

When symptoms of gastroparesis occur, treatment should be sought because food that stays in the stomach too long can ferment, causing bacterial growth, or may harden into a solid lump, called a bezoar. Slow digestion of food will affect diabetics insofar as diabetic medications may hit their peak effectiveness too soon, wearing off by the time the food is finally digested and causing high blood sugar levels (Roberts, 2001). (See Table 4.3).

Dumping syndrome. Often following stomach surgery for obesity or peptic ulcer, dumping syndrome "is believed to be caused by the rapid entry of hyperosmolar liquids into the intestine and is characterized by symptoms such as nausea, vomiting, diarrhea, diaphoresis, palpitations, tachycardia, lightheadedness, and flushing that occur while eating or shortly after" (Porth, 1998, p. 728). It is often followed in about 2 hours by an episode of hypoglycemia, resulting from the rapid absorption of glucose, which acts as a stimulus for insulin release by the B cells of the pancreas. With treatment however, the symptoms of dumping syndrome subside over time.

Overall for both gastroparesis and dumping syndrome the role of glucose plays an important role. The research of Rayner, Samsom, Jones, and Horowitz (2001) indicates that acute hyperglycemia induced by an intravenous glucose infusion slows the emptying of nutrient-containing liquid and solid meals. Conversely, gastric emptying of both solids and liquids is accelerated during insulin-induced hypoglycemia.

GENERAL NURSING CARE

Gastroparesis. Nursing diagnoses for the patient with gastroparesis include: knowledge deficit related to the disease process, chronic pain related to

TABLE 4.3   Possible Complications of Gastroparesis

Complication	Description and Treatment
Bezoars	Food hardened into solid lumps due to stomach stasis. May cause massive infection when untreated or not resolved. Treatment: antibiotics (Erythromycin) and/or removal by endoscopy or surgery.
Hyperglycemia in diabetics	Slow digestion of food may precipitate high blood sugar because diabetic medications may peak too soon. Treatment: smaller and more frequent doses of insulin.

gastric immobility, altered nutrition and altered fluids related to gastric immobility, effective management of therapeutic regime for individual and family, and potential for infection related to withholding of stomach contents.

Nursing care centers upon the understanding of the older adult regarding his/her disease process. Discomfort related to gas and bloating is most upsetting to the patient and can be managed with medications and food selection. For acute and severe gastric immobility it may be necessary to supplement the client's diet with tube feedings or TPN to maintain nutritional and fluid stability. In less severe and chronic cases, manipulation of the diet into 6 small feedings is helpful to ensure adequate intake. As stasis of stomach contents can ultimately lead to the formation of bezoars, for which antibiotic therapy is necessary, or even extraction by endoscopy, watching for signs and symptoms of infection, and treating the possible side effects of antibiotic therapy (stomach upset, diarrhea) may be necessary. Because the condition may be chronic, understanding the therapeutic regimen and following it is imperative for clients and the nurse assists clients in implementing gastro interventions for their holistic health. If the client is diabetic, the regimen must include alterations in diet and insulin therapy.

Dumping syndrome. Nursing diagnoses for the older adult with dumping syndrome include: knowledge deficit related to the disease process, altered nutrition related to increased gastric mobility, and diarrhea related to rapid gastric emptying. Nursing care centers on educating the client regarding the cause of the dumping syndrome and how to prevent it. Diet therapy is essential in preventing the symptoms of hypoglycemia, and medications taken to thicken oral liquids (thereby holding them longer in the stomach), may be helpful to clients. If patients are experiencing severe diarrhea, interventions may include the decreasing of oral fluids and the taking of antidiarrhea medications.

INTERVENTIONS, TREATMENTS, ALTERNATIVE TREATMENTS

Gastroparesis. Three questions should be considered in the management of the older patient with gastroparesis: Is the condition acute or chronic? Does the patient have a systemic disorder such as neuropathy or myopathy? What is the patient's state of hydration and nutrition? The principal methods of management include correction of dehydration and nutritional deficiencies, the use of prokinetic and antiemetic medications, and the suppression of bacterial overgrowth. Decompression of the stomach and surgery are necessary only in patients with severe motility problems (Camilleri, 1998).

Correction of dehydration, and electrolyte and nutritional depletion, is particularly important during acute exacerbations of gastroparesis. Nutrition is tailored to each patient according to individual depletions in trace elements and dietary constituents. Dietary measures include low-fiber and low-fat caloric supplements that contain iron, folate, calcium, and vitamins D, K, and B_{12} (Camilleri, 1998). Patients who have intense symptoms of nausea and vomiting, such as often seen in severe diabetics, may have need of parenteral or enteral nutrition. If a feeding tube is necessary, a jejunostomy tube is recommended as nutrients are placed directly in the small intestine, bypassing the stomach altogether. In patients who tolerate oral feedings, fatty and high-fiber foods should be avoided, and six small meals should be eaten each day rather than three (NIDDK/NIH, 1999). Liquid meals are recommended, especially if blood glucose levels are unstable. (See Table 4.4).

Prokinetic medications, like metaclopramide (Reglan) in doses of 10 to 20 mg given up to four times a day, is being used to increase the sensitivity to acetylcholine, resulting in increased motility of the upper GI tract and relaxation of the pyloric sphincter. This increases gastric emptying time and improves the gastroparesis condition.

Erythromycin, a macrolide antibiotic that stimulates motilin receptors partly through a cholinergic mechanism, results in the dumping of nondi-

TABLE 4.4 Management of Gastroparesis

Correct Dehydration, Electrolyte, or Nutritional Depletion	1. Low-fiber, low-fat caloric supplements 2. 6 small meals per day rather than 3 3. Liquid meals if blood glucose levels are unstable 4. Parenteral or enteral nutritional support
Medications	1. G.I. motility drugs to promote movement and emptying of stomach Metoclopramide (Reglan) 2. Antibiotics to clear and prevent bezoars Erythromycin 3. Antiemetics to reduce nausea & vomiting
Decompression and/or Gastric Surgery	1. Nasogastric intubations—relieves abdominal distention and bloating, removes stagnant gastric fluids 2. Venting enterostomy—relieves abdominal distention and bloating 3. Partial or complete gastrectomy—to remove sections of stomach with permanent stasis following gastric surgery

gestible and digestible solids from the stomach. Erythromycin lactobionate at a dosage of 3 to 6 mg/kg every eight hours clears bezoars from the stomach in patients with diabetic gastroparesis (Camilleri). However, the effect of oral erythromycin appears to be restricted by tachyphylaxis, and this treatment is considered ineffective after two weeks. Bezoars not responsive to antibiotic therapy may necessitate removal through endoscopy.

For treatment of nausea and vomiting associated with gastroparesis, standard antiemetics can be used in combination with prokinetic agents for symptom relief. These include medications such as diphenhydramine (Benadryl) and trifluoperazine (Stelazine), or metaclopramide (Reglan).

Decompression may be used for patients whose gastroparesis is accompanied by severe pseudo-obstruction of the bowel. Venting enterostomy can assist in relieving abdominal distention and bloating. There are enteral tubes which function for both aspiration and feeding using the same apparatus. Access to the small intestine may also provide a way to deliver nutrients by the enteral route (Camilleri, 1998).

Surgical treatment should be considered whenever the motility disorder is localized to a portion of the gut that can be resected. For example, complete gastrectomy may be necessary for patients with complete stasis syndrome following gastric surgery (Camilleri, 1998).

If the cause of gastroparesis is related to diabetes, the primary treatment goal is to regain control of blood glucose levels. Treatments include insulin, oral medications, and dietary changes regarding calories as well as fat and fiber intake. Recommendations regarding insulin therapy include taking insulin more often, taking insulin after eating instead of before, checking blood levels frequently after eating, and administering insulin whenever necessary. Some physicians may recommend two injections of intermediate insulin every day, and also increase the number of injections of a fast-acting insulin as needed according to blood glucose levels obtained in frequent monitoring. Lispro insulin (Humalog), a newer insulin, is a quick-acting insulin that appears to be advantageous for people with gastroparesis. It starts working within 5 to 15 minutes after injection and peaks after 1 to 2 hours, thus lowering blood glucose levels after eating almost twice as fast as the slower-acting regular insulin (NIH, 1999).

Dumping syndrome. Management primarily includes patient education with regard to avoiding high-nutrient liquid drinks, and fluids with meals. Possibly guar gum or pectin may be given to retard liquid emptying. On rare occasions, medications such as subcutaneuous octreotide (Sandostatin) (50 to 100 mg) may be prescribed to be taken 15 minutes before meals (Camilleri, 1998). Octreotide is a potent growth hormone similar to somatostatin and is currently being investigated for its usefulness in dealing with the effects of dumping syndrome (Mosby's Nursing Drug Reference, 2002). Dicyclomine hydrochloride (Bentyl), an antispasmodic, may also be prescribed to help delay gastric emptying time.

Dumping Syndrome treatment also consists of limiting the diet to small frequent feedings, which are taken without liquids and which are low in simple sugars, because they are the most osmotically active parts of the diet. The symptoms of Dumping Syndrome usually diminish with time, and may be dissipated within three months (Roberts, 2001). (See Table 4.5).

Alternative measures may be suggested as helpful in the treatment of gastroparesis or Dumping Syndrome, for example in promoting digestion, or relieving diarrhea. It is believed that yoga exercises can enhance digestion and help the pancreas and liver function more normally, thereby regulating blood sugar levels. Since almost 20% of persons with Type I diabetes may develop gastroparesis, these exercises may be of interest to clients as a complementary therapy. Yoga exercises that are helpful for gastric health are described by Dr. Monro and Dr. Nagendra in the popular alternative medicine book entitled *New Choices in Natural Healings* (Gottlieb, 1995). The following exercise would be easy to teach the older adult: Stand with your feet spread apart approximately to shoulder-width. Place your hands

TABLE 4.5   Management of Dumping Syndrome

Assess for signs of dumping syndrome	Early Symptoms (within 30 minute of eating): Flushing, diaphoresis, weakness, dizziness, faintness, abdominal pain and distention, increased bowel sounds, diarrhea, irregular pulse, hypotension Late Symptoms ($1\frac{1}{2}$ to 3 hours postprandial): Hypoglycemic-like reaction similar to the signs and symptoms listed above
Teach patient ways to prevent "dumping syndrome"	Eat small frequent meals Avoid simple carbohydrates (sugar) in diet Increase protein and fat (to tolerance) in diet Omit fluids with meals, take fluids 1 hour before or 2 hours after eating Eat slowly and chew food well Lie down 20 to 30 minutes after eating
Medications	Dicyclomine hydrochloride (Bentyl)—antispasmodic to delay emptying time Octreotide (Sandostatin)—investigational drug to retard liquid emptying

on your knees and bend forward. Exhale through your mouth until all your breath is gone. Now expand your chest, and tighten your abdominal muscles so that you form a hollow space in your abdomen. Remain in this position until you feel the need to breathe, then relax and inhale slowly. The next step is abdominal pumping. Release your stomach muscles back to their normal position, and then suck in the abdominal muscles again. Pump your abdomen in and out until you experience the need to breathe. Release slowly and breathe normally. Repeat the entire exercise three times.

To avoid dehydration during a bout of diarrhea, Dr. Lad (Gottlieb, 1995) suggests drinking water with honey, lime juice, and salt. He says to add one teaspoon of honey, one teaspoon of lime juice, and a pinch of salt to a pint of warm or room temperature water and sip it throughout the day.

HEALTH PROMOTION AND QUALITY OF LIFE ISSUES

For most patients gastroparesis and dumping syndrome are not life threatening. The good news with dumping syndrome is that it usually lasts only a few months at most! Depending on its causes, gastroparesis is usually a chronic condition that can be managed and allows the client an acceptable quality of life.

Health promotion efforts can only assist the client in maintaining a healthier lifestyle. A diet which is balanced yet within the parameters of the associated condition (i.e., low fiber for gastroparesis and low sugar for dumping syndrome) can assist in overall health and well-being. Vitamin supplements, such as one multivitamin a day at least, are recommended.

Exercise benefits the entire body especially aiding circulation and control of weight. Walking at least 15 minutes a day can improve appetite and relieve stress. Stress and anxiety only heighten feelings of discomfort in gastroparesis and may contribute to episodes of diarrhea in the client with dumping syndrome.

For the client with severe gastroparesis to the point of the entire stomach being paralyzed, surgical removal of the stomach may be necessary. Continual tube feedings may be required for nutritional support for which the question of quality of life may surface. It would seem that absent other complications or debilitating conditions, a client can experience an acceptable quality of life despite the need for continuous nutritional support. The client retains the right to refuse nutritional support, of course, and counseling must be given to ensure that the client realizes he/she is choosing death. With the caring support of health professionals, family, and friends, it is hoped that the client would not experience the need for such a drastic measure. In addition to the above interventions, the client's level of depression must be assessed, and treated with antidepressants, if necessary.

The possibility of depression or despair, and feelings of hopelessness or discomfort indicate the need for therapy to bring meaning into the person's life. The client must come to accept the reason for the suffering and limitations brought about by this chronic condition. This presents a possibility for teaching centering, guided imagery, or relaxation techniques which promote peace and increase the client's sensitivity to spiritual realities. Perhaps if the client is religious, a leader or member of the religious community may help the client through prayer and spiritual support.

HOME MANAGEMENT AND SELF-CARE ISSUES

Home management centers upon proper diet, timing of meals, attention to portion size, and fluid regulation. Older adults and their families need to understand what foods are included within their recommended diets, such as low fiber or high protein. Printed dietary instructions would be helpful to most clients. Diabetics should consult with their nurse practitioner or physician regarding the regulation of insulin, since both hypoglycemia and hyperglycemia can occur with dumping syndrome and gastroparesis. Difficulty with self-care should not be an issue if the patient is otherwise independent in their activities of daily living and is mentally functional. However, if tube feedings are necessary for the patient with gastroparesis, the client and his/her significant others must be taught care of the feeding tube, skin care, management of the pump, and handling of the liquid nutrient in order to prevent occlusion of the tube, or infection.

FOLLOW-UP CARE

Follow-up care with the elderly client should include evaluation for possible weight loss and dehydration. It may be helpful to ask the client to keep a dietary journal, so that it is possible to discuss strengths and weaknesses regarding eating patterns and the responses encountered after eating certain foods or drinks. A hematocrit and electrolytes profile may be needed in the presence of severe nausea, vomiting, or diarrhea. Medication use should be evaluated and prescriptions renewed as necessary. In the client with dumping syndrome any episodes of hypoglycemic reactions should be reviewed with the client, especially the factors preceding it, to determine if reinforcement of teaching is necessary. In general, all signs and symptoms experienced by the client should be discussed to regulate medication as needed and to provide psychological support and caring.

CONCLUSION

The older adult may find certain foods "difficult to digest" and may experience loss of appetite, or early satiety, or feel uncomfortable with bloating after eating. Gastroparesis, a sluggishness in the motility of stomach muscles causing food to remain longer in the stomach, may be the cause. Understanding the pathology can help the client alter his/her eating patterns, thus reducing some of the signs and symptoms. Although less common, dumping syndrome may be experienced in the older adult who has undergone gastric surgery. The best management for this syndrome is most commonly found in teaching the client to eat smaller, more frequent meals, and to omit fluids with meals.

REFERENCES

Birrer, R. B. (2002). Irritable bowel syndrome. *Disease-A-Month, 48*(2), page 1 05–143.

Burrell, L., Gerlach, M., & Pless, B. (1997). *Adult nursing: Acute and community care.* Stamford, CT: Appleton & Lange.

Camilleri, M. (1998). Gastro XIV, Gastrointestinal motility disorders. In D. C. Dale & D. D. Federmann (Eds.), *Scientific American medicine.* New York: Scientific American, Inc.

D'Arrigo, T. (1999). Solving a gut-wrenching problem. *Diabetes Forecast, 52*(8), 81–83.

Dorland's Illustrated Medical Dictionary. (1994). Philadelphia: W. B. Saunders Company.

Gottlieb, B. (1995). *New choices in natural healing.* Emmaus, PA: Rodale Press, Inc.

Mosby's Nursing Drug Reference. (2002). St. Louis: Mosby.

National Digestive Diseases Information Clearinghouse (NIDDK) (1999). NIH Publication No. 99-4348. Retrieved from *http://www.niddk.nih.gov/health/digest/pubs/gastro/gastro.htm*

Porth, C. M. (1998). *Pathophysiology: Concepts of altered health states.* New York: Lippincott.

Rayner, C. K., Samsom, M., Jones, K. L., & Horowitz, M. (2001). Relationships of upper gastrointestinal motor and sensory function with glycemic control. *Diabetes Care, 24*(2), 371.

Roberts, S. S. (2001). When stomachs get sluggish. *Diabetes Forecast, 54*(11), 24–25.

Helicobacter Pylori and Ulcers

Phyllis J. Atkinson

The bacterium Helicobacter pylori (H. pylori) was discovered in 1982 by Dr. Barry Marshall. Studies have been conducted around the world since then. The discovery of H. pylori changed the concept of peptic ulcer disease (PUD) etiology, previously thought to strictly be a chronic, acid-related condition. The discovery of H. pylori also changed the concept of care and management of PUD.

H. pylori is common in the United States and is also one of the most common bacteria in the world. Approximately two-thirds of the world's population is infected with H. pylori (CDC). About 20 percent of people less than 40 years old and half of those over 60 are infected with H. pylori. Most infected people do not develop ulcers; however, most ulcers are the result of H. pylori infection.

H. pylori is more common in older adults, African Americans, Latinos, and lower socioeconomic groups. It is less common in more affluent Caucasians. H. pylori is most commonly found in countries where stomach cancer is prevalent. These countries include Colombia, China, Japan, Peru, and Scotland.

DEFINITIONS

H. pylori is a gram-negative, flagellated, spiral-shaped bacterium found in the gastric mucous layer or clinging to the epithelial lining of the stomach.

The genus Helicobacter is composed of at least 25 species that share common properties and characteristics. It is predominantly acquired in childhood. It is associated with lifelong chronic gastritis and may cause other gastroduodenal disorders and their complications. H. pylori is believed to be the leading cause of duodenal and gastric ulcers. H. pylori causes more than 90% of duodenal ulcers and up to 80% of gastric ulcers (CDC, 2002). The World Health Organization has defined H. pylori as a Group 1 carcinogen.

An ulcer is a sore on the lining of the stomach or duodenum. Peptic ulcers are common. Approximately 25 million Americans (10%) suffer from PUD at some point in their lifetime (CDC, 2002). Hospitalization, morbidity, and mortality rates from PUD are higher for older adults (Borum, 2002). A peptic ulcer is referred to either as gastric, duodenal or esophageal, depending on its location (Grzelak, 2000).

ETIOLOGY

The prevalence of H. pylori infections increases with age. Almost all patients infected with H. pylori develop gastritis and 15% develop PUD (Borum). Why H. pylori does not cause ulcers in every infected person is unknown. There is a strong correlation between H. pylori gastritis and duodenal ulcers. In the absence of the use of nonsteroidal antiinflammatory drugs (NSAIDs) and Zollinger-Ellison Syndrome, H. pylori is believed to be the prerequisite for the occurrence of almost all duodenal ulcers.

It is not clear how people contract H. pylori. Nor is it clear why some patients become symptomatic and others do not. How it is transmitted is also not clear. It is thought to be orally transmitted. Some believe it is transmitted orally by fecal matter in contaminated food or water. Another theory is that H. pylori is transmitted from the stomach to the mouth through gastroesophageal reflux with the bacterium then being transmitted through oral contact.

The incubation period of an acute H. pylori infection is from one to seven days and may or may not be followed by dyspeptic syndrome. The symptoms are estimated to last for approximately one week, and then disappear whether or not the H. pylori has been eliminated (McManus, 2000).

H. pylori has been associated with iron deficiency anemia, salivary gland mucosal-associated-lymphoid-type (MALT) lymphomas, as well as gastric carcinoma. Those infected with H. pylori have a 2 to 6-fold increased risk of developing gastric cancer and MALT lymphoma. Gastric cancer is the second most common cancer worldwide (CDC).

Risk factors for H. pylori include smoking, alcohol use, poor nutrition, genetic factors such as Japanese descent, and psychological stress. Patients with a history of achlorhydria (an abnormal condition with an absence of hydrochloric acid in the gastric juices) and pernicious anemia are at an even greater risk for the development of gastric cancer. Gastric cancer usually occurs in mid to late life after a long exposure to the H. pylori infection.

After menopause peptic ulcers occur as frequently in women as they do men. Risk factors for the development of PUD include the use of NSAIDs. Other risk factors include the ingestion of products that can increase hydrochloric acid secretion such as milk, caffeinated beverages, smoking, and alcohol. A condition called Zollinger-Ellison Syndrome (severe peptic ulceration, gastric hypersecretion, elevated serum gastrin, and gastrinona of the pancreas or duodenum) as well as being infected with H. pylori increase the incidence of peptic ulcers. Individuals with Type O blood are also at greater risk for the development of peptic ulcers.

There are differences in the risk factors associated with gastric ulcers versus those with duodenal ulcers. The risk factors for gastric ulcers include H. pylori, gastritis, alcohol, smoking, NSAIDs, and stress. The risks factors for duodenal ulcers include H. pylori, Type O blood group, chronic obstructive lung disease, chronic renal failure, alcohol, smoking, cirrhosis, and stress.

PATHOLOGY

The exact pathogenesis of H. pylori is unknown. The stomach is protected from its own gastric juice by a thick layer of mucus that covers the stomach lining. The integrity of the mucus-bicarbonate barrier is prostaglandin-dependent. Older adults have a decrease in prostaglandin concentrations in the stomach and duodenum. H. pylori makes its way to the protective mucous lining where its spiral shape helps it burrow through the lining.

H. pylori is able to survive in the acidity of the stomach because it secretes the enzyme, urease, that neutralizes the acid. Urease converts urea (large amount in stomach) into bicarbonate and ammonia (both strong bases). Ammonia neutralizes gastric acid and is toxic to gastric epithelial cells. The conversion of urea produces a cloud of acid neutralizing chemicals around the H. pylori, protecting it from the acid in the stomach.

The body's natural defenses have not been able to reach H. pylori in the mucus lining of the stomach. The immune system responds to H. pylori by sending white cells, killer T cells, and other infection fighting agents. These agents can't seem to reach the H. pylori, primarily because it is not easy for them to get through the mucus lining. The immune system continues to keep sending defense agents, which, when they die, release superoxide radicals on the stomach lining cells. H. pylori feeds on this and within a few days, gastritis and in some cases peptic ulcer develops. Some theorize it is not the H. pylori itself that causes peptic ulcer but the inflammation of the stomach lining. The effect of aging on the immunologic factors that may protect against H. pylori have not been determined.

The clinical syndrome of acute H. pylori infection appears to be associated with epigastric cramping pain, nausea, vomiting, flatulence, malaise, and halitosis. Many patients remain asymptomatic (McManus, 2000).

A peptic ulcer is caused by the erosion of a circumscribed area of mucous membrane. The erosion may extend as deeply as the muscle layers or through the muscle to the peritoneum. Peptic ulcers generally occur alone but can occur in multiples (Grzelak, 2000).

When food is ingested the body responds by binding acetylcholine, gastrin, and histamine to specific receptors which stimulate the parietal cells in the fundus of the stomach to secrete hydrochloric acid. With the assistance of the hydrogen-potassium adenosine triphosphatase pump, the parietal cells transport the hydrochloric acid to the stomach lumen. Pepsinogen is secreted by the chief cells in the stomach. In the presence of hydrochloric acid pepsinogen is converted to pepsin, which assists in the breakdown of food. The gastroduodenal lining is protected by a mucous barrier which is secreted by the duodenal cells in the gastric epithelium (Grzelak, 2000).

Peptic ulcers occur mainly in the gastroduodenal mucosa as the tissue there cannot withstand the digestive action of hydrochloric acid and pepsin. Erosion occurs in the presence of either increased concentration or activity of acid-pepsin, or to decreased resistance of the mucosa. When the mucosa is damaged it cannot secrete enough mucus to act as a barrier against hydrochloric acid. NSAIDs inhibit the secretion of mucus (Grzelak, 2000).

Duodenal ulcer may be related to acid hypersecretion. The pain associated with duodenal ulcer will often awaken the patient between midnight and 3:00 A.M. It is often relieved by antacids, eating, or even vomiting.

Gastric ulcer is associated with normal or reduced rates of acid production. Older adults have reduced acid production and therefore have higher incidences of gastric ulcers. Food may precipitate or worsen pain.

Gastric ulcers in older adults may be located more proximally in the stomach (Borum, 2002). Duodenal ulcers may be larger in older adults with ulcers > 2 cm often reported in older adults. Bleeding from duodenal ulcers occur more frequently in older adults (Borum, 2002).

Untreated gastric ulcers caused by H. pylori are significantly linked to the development of gastric carcinomas over time.

GENERAL NURSING CARE

Nursing care should focus on the appropriate assessment of potential risks factors, changes in stools, vomiting, and recent stressful events. Always question patients about the use of over-the-counter medications. Self-treatment with antacids could indicate a potential ulcer that may otherwise not be recognized.

Nursing care should also focus on the prevention of complications that often accompany PUD. These complications include hemorrhage, perforation, penetration, and pyloric obstruction (Grzelak, 2000).

Patient education should focus on the disease process, the purpose of diagnostic testing, the purpose and side effects of medication, and potential drug interactions. The importance of stress reduction and smoking cessation should also be emphasized (Astarita, 1999).

It is imperative to assure proper medication compliance for the treatment of H. pylori and peptic ulcers. Patients need to be educated on the importance of medication compliance. The use of a medication compliance device such as a mediplanner may be useful.

NURSING DIAGNOSES AND PLAN OF CARE

Some of the nursing diagnoses that are applicable to the patient with either H. pylori or PUD include:

- Pain related to the effect of gastric acid secretion on damaged tissue
- Anxiety related to coping with an acute illness
- Altered nutrition related to changes in diet
- Knowledge deficit about prevention of symptoms and management of the condition (Grzelak, 2000)

Goals of care should include relieving any pain, reducing anxiety, maintaining adequate nutrition, and accelerating ulcer healing. Other goals include educating about the management and prevention of ulcer recurrence as well as avoiding complications.

INTERVENTIONS, TREATMENTS, ALTERNATIVE TREATMENT

NSAIDs should be discontinued. The use of alcohol, tobacco and caffeine should be eliminated.

Pain from PUD can be relieved by the elimination of the causative factors mentioned above. In addition, the administration of prescribed medications will relieve pain.

Reduction of anxiety can be achieved by teaching relaxation techniques, biofeedback, hypnosis, or behavioral modification. Psychological counseling may also be needed and should be encouraged if needed.

Elimination of H. pylori is indicated in patients with proven peptic ulcers. There is no therapy that is 100% effective in treating H. pylori. Currently, H. pylori peptic ulcers are treated with drugs that kill the bacteria, reduce stomach acid, and protect the stomach lining. Antibiotics are used to kill the bacteria. Antibiotics such as Meronidazole, Tetracycline, Clarithromycin, and Amoxicillin may also be used to treat H. pylori. H_2 blockers (ranitidine, famotidine, nizatidine, and cimetidine) and proton pump inhibitors (omeprazole, lansoprazole, and rabeprazole) may be used to treat H. pylori peptic ulcers. Both H_2 inhibitors and PPIs are acid-suppressing drugs.

H_2 blockers work by blocking histamine, which stimulates acid secretion. It usually takes a few weeks before the pain of the ulcer is relieved after therapy is started.

PPIs suppress acid protection by halting the mechanism that pumps the acid into the stomach. For years H_2 blockers and PPIs have been prescribed as monotherapy for the treatment of ulcers; however, used alone they will not eradicate H. pylori and therefore do not cure H. pylori ulcers.

Treatment should include combination of antibiotics, H_2 blockers, and PPIs. The bismuth triple therapy has been FDA approved in the United States. Bismuth subsalicylate, a component of Pepto-Bismol, is used to protect the stomach lining form acid.

Due to antibiotic resistance seen in different regions the type of antibiotic used may vary. Clarithromycin is more resistant in older adults as well as those living in the Northeast and Mid-Atlantic regions. At present the recommended therapy is a 2-week course of treatment referred to as triple therapy. It includes two antibiotics to kill the bacteria and either a PPI or

H_2 blocker. Triple therapy reduces ulcer symptoms, kills the bacteria, and prevents ulcer recurrence in more than 90 percent of patients.

Triple therapy can be difficult for some patients because it often includes taking 20 medications a day. Moshkowitz and colleagues found that a one-week treatment of triple therapy consisting of omeprazole, Clarithromycin and tinidazole was effective in eradicating H. pylori in older adults.

The unpleasant side effects of the antibiotics can results in noncompliance. Some of these side effects include diarrhea, nausea/vomiting, a metallic taste in the mouth, dizziness, headache, and yeast infections in women.

The Bismuth quadruple therapy is also used. This includes two weeks of quadruple therapy, using two antibiotics, a PPI and an H_2 blocker. It is more difficult to follow.

Many other antibiotics have shown promising results in clinical studies but are not yet FDA approved. Some of these include Furazolidone, Asithromycin, and Ciprofloxacin.

In patients who do not respond to drug treatment, surgery such as gastretomy or partial gastrectomy is an option.

HEALTH PROMOTION AND QUALITY OF LIFE ISSUES

There is no clear etiology of how H. pylori spreads, so prevention is difficult. Researchers are working on a vaccine to prevent the infection.

HOME MANAGEMENT AND SELF-CARE ISSUES

Education as to preventive measures to prevent H. pylori include encouragement of good hand washing before eating and after using the bathroom, as well as avoid eating food not properly prepared, and drinking safe, clean water.

Medications need to be reviewed with the patient, including proper administration as well as potential side effects. Causative factors need to be reviewed and their elimination encouraged. Proper diet should be stressed. Patients should also be educated as to signs and symptoms to report. If needed, the patient should be encouraged to attend smoking cessation classes.

FOLLOW-UP CARE

Patients should be encouraged to be retested for H. pylori after the treatment; however, patients may remain seropostive for more than three years after treatment. Patients should be encouraged to return for follow-up in 10 to 14 days after treatment is initiated, at the end of treatment for symptom assessment, and again in four to six weeks for reassessment and retesting for H. pylori eradication (Astarita, 1999). If an NSAID user tested negative for H. pylori they should be referred to a gastroenterologist for endoscopic evaluation prior to treatment (Astarita, 1999).

Recurrence after treatment of an ulcer is not likely if the causative factors have been eradicated. Smoking and alcohol cessation should be strongly encouraged since both increase the likelihood of recurrence. Patients need to be encouraged to report all possible signs/symptoms of recurrence.

After anti-ulcer therapy is initiated the patient should follow-up in 10 to 14 days and again in four to six weeks to assess symptoms. If symptoms remain, the patient should be referred to gastroenterologist for endoscopic evaluation (Astarita, 1999). Prior to beginning NSAID therapy, H. pylori testing should be completed.

REFERENCES

Astrarita, T. (1999, December). Update in peptic ulcer disease management. *Patient Care for the Nurse Practitioner*, 39–52.

Borum, M. (2002). Gastric disorders. Retrieved from *http://www.merck.com/pubs/ mm_geritrics/sec13/ch106.htm*

CDC (2002). Helicobacter pylori and peptic ulcer disease. Retrieved from *http:// www.cdc.gov/ulcer/md.htm*

Chey, W., & Marshall, B. (2002). Treatment of Helicobacter pylori. Retrieved from *http://www.helico.com/newsite/trsum.html*

Grzelak, G. (2000). Management of patients with gastric and duodenal disorders. In S. Smeltzer & B. Bare (Eds.), *Brunner & Suddarth's textbook of medical surgical nursing* (9th ed., pp 857–868). Philadelphia: J. B. Lippincott Company.

The Helicobacter Pylori Foundation (2002). About Helicobacter pylori. Retrieved from *http://www.helico.com/newsite/aboutpylori.html*

Moshkowitz, M., Brill, S., Konikoff, F. M., Arber, N., & Halpern, Z. (1999). *Journal of the American Geriatric Society, 47*(6), 720–722.

Meyer, J., Silliman, N., & Wang, W. (2002). Risk factors for helicobacter pylori resistance in the United States: The surveillance of H. pylori antimocrobial resistance partnership(SHARP) study, 1993–1999. *Annals of Internal Medicine, 136*, 13–24.

McManus, T. (2000). Helicobacter pylori: An emerging infectious disease. *The Nurse Practitioner, 25*(8), 40–53.

NIDDK/NIH. (2002). H. pylori and peptic ulcer. Retrieved from *http://www.niddk.nih. gov/health/digest/pubs/hpylori/hpylori.html*

Uemura, N., Yamamoto, S., Yamaguchi, S., Yamakido, M., Taniyama, K., Sasaki, N., & Schlemper, R. J. (2001). Helicobacter pylori infection and the development of gastric cancer. *The New England Journal of Medicine, 345*(11), 784–789.

Walling, A. (June, 2000). Antibiotic treatment of patients with H. pylori. Retrieved from *http://www.americanfamilyphysician.com*

—6—

Bacterial, Viral, and Parasitic Infections of the Colon

Sue E. Meiner

Infections of the colon include bacterial, viral, and less frequently parasitic. Virusal and fungal infections are often associated with immunosuppressed persons, very ill older adults, and persons with weakening comorbidities. While most infections are self-limiting, dysentery with severe diarrhea and sepsis can be a serious illness and can lead to a life-threatening situation. Factors that influence the susceptibility to infection include age, gastric acid levels, intestinal motility, colonization resistance, and immune state. Advanced age plays a major role.

Elderly residents in long-term-care facilities, day-care facilities, and hospitals are especially susceptible to infections of the colon. One such nosocomial infection is Clostridium difficile colitis. Another bacterium that is especially dangerous in older adults is Salmonella. This infection can often have a virulent course especially when comorbidities are present as is often present in the frail elderly (Nassar, Hasan, & Gregg, 2000).

Viral and parasitic infections can present with watery diarrhea-leading to rapid dehydration. The rotaviruses, adenoviruses, astroviruses, caliciviruses, and Norwalk-like viruses are the most common diarrhea-causing agents in viral gastroenteritis in the United States. Parasites that cause diarrhea include Giardia lamblia, Entamoeba histolytica, Cryptosporidium parvum, and Cyclospora cayetanensis (Nassar, Hasan, & Gregg, 2000; Richter, 2000). This chapter will present information on the clinical presentation of the bacterial, viral, and parasitic causes of infectious gastroenteritis. Recommendations for nursing care and treatment are presented. This information is instructive but does not replace the advice or recommendations of a primary care provider with specific information relevant to a patient.

DEFINITIONS

Diarrhea can be defined as the passage of three or more unformed bowel movements in a 24-hour period. Labels such as acute, chronic, or persistent are based upon the time frame of the occurrence. The majority of infectious causes of diarrhea are mild and self-limited over a three- to five-day period. Diarrhea that lasts less than 14 days is termed acute diarrhea. Persistent diarrhea is identified as lasting between two and four weeks. Diarrhea lasting over four weeks is identified as chronic diarrhea.

Specifically, diarrhea is characterized by increased stool water content, which may be a consequence of increased fluid secretion, decreased water absorption, or altered bowel motility. A combination of mechanisms is also possible. Increased fluid secretion can be stimulated by an inflammatory process, hormones, or enterotoxins. Decreased reabsorption of fluid occurs primarily with abnormalities of the bowel mucosa. Increased bowel motility reduces the fecal contact time with the bowel mucosa, which limits fluid reabsorption. An example of this mechanism is with the use of laxatives that create limited fecal contact time with the bowel mucosa leading to stool evacuation (Richter, 2000).

ETIOLOGY

Intestinal infections are the single largest cause of morbidity and mortality around the world. Unsanitary living conditions and improper food handling and hygienic practices are the major determinants of exposure to pathogens. Patterns of illnesses with predominant diarrhea vary significantly with climate and seasonal variations. Nearly all infective agents are transmitted by the fecal-oral route. While fatalities are rare, gastroenteritis and acute diarrhea account for 1.5% of hospitalizations of adults in the United States.

The Centers for Disease Control and Prevention (CDC) identified the Norwalk virus to be responsible for more than 40% of viral gastroenteritis among adults in a five year study (National Center for Infectious Diseases, 2001). Viral outbreaks can be the result of food-borne, water-borne, or person-to-person contamination.

PATHOLOGY

Microbial factors include the effects of bacterial toxins and their adhesion abilities. Bacterial toxins are classified into three types: neurotoxins, entero-toxins, and cytotoxins. Bacterial toxins responsible for producing disease are classified as neurotoxins. Examples of neurotoxins are Staphylococcus and Clostridium botulinum. Large fluid secretions from the intestinal tract are caused by enterotoxins, such as Vibrio cholerae, Salmonella, Shigella, Escherichia coli. Cytotoxins damage the muscosa. Examples of cytotoxins are Clostridium difficile, Clostridium perfringens, and Escherichia coli. See Table 6.1 for a list of common pathogens responsible for colon infections.

Clostridium difficile (C. diff.) colitis is associated with antibiotic therapy. Pharmacotherapy with a broad-spectrum antibiotic predisposes the older person to disruption of the normal bacterial flora in the colon. When colonization by C. diff. occurs, a release of toxins follows. This release causes a pseudomembranous colitis due to the mucosal damage and inflam-mation. While other antibiotics can cause C. diff., the broad-spectrum

TABLE 6.1   Common Pathogens in Colon Infections

General Population	Sexually Transmitted	Immunocompromised
Shigella	Campylobacter	Salmonella
Salmonella	Shigella	Shigella
Campylobacter	Neisseria gonorrhea	Clostridium difficile
Clostridium difficile	Chlamydia trachomatis	Clostridium septicum
Enterohemorrhagic E. coli	Herpes simplex virus type 2	Mycobacterium-avium intracellular
Enteroinvasive E. coli	Entamoeba histolytica	Cytomegalovirus
Aeromonas		Herpes simplex virus
Yersinia enterocolitica		Adenovirus
Vibrio parahaemolyticus		Candida albicans
Entamoeba histolytica		Aspergillus

antibiotics given for gram-negative enteric bacteria are the most frequently targeted as the responsible agent. Penicillins and cephalosporins are examples of the most commonly prescribed medicines associated with C. diff. enteric infections. The infection is manifested by diarrhea that is mild to moderate and sometimes accompanied by lower abdominal cramping (Porth, 1998).

The more severe form of C. diff. colitis is characterized by an adherent inflammatory membrane overlying the areas of mucosal injury. It is a life-threatening form of the disease. Persons with the disease are acutely ill, with lethargy, fever, tachycardia, abdominal pain and distention, and dehydration. Patients can be contaminated from environmental surfaces, shared instrumentation, hospital personnel, and infected roommates. The smooth muscle tone of the colon may be lost, resulting in toxic dilation of the colon. The bowel may become perforated if prompt therapy is not initiated. Antibiotic therapy must be discontinued immediately when these symptoms are assessed (Barbut & Petit, 2001; Porth, 1998).

Escherichia coli (O157:H7) is strongly associated with epidemic and sporadic colitis. Public awareness was heightened when a national fast-food chain was identified with undercooked hamburger and the resulting E. coli enteric infection of its customers. The specific strain of E. coli (O157:H7) is found in feces and in contaminated milk of otherwise healthy dairy and beef cattle. It has been found in other meats such as pork, poultry, and lamb. While person-to-person transmission is possible, undercooked meat is more likely to be the agent of transmission. Symptoms can vary from none to acute, nonbloody diarrhea, hemorrhagic colitis, hemolytic-uremic syndrome, and thrombotic thrombocytopenic purpura. Often beginning with watery diarrhea, the disease progresses, if unchecked, to include bloody diarrhea with fever. The diarrhea can last between three and seven days or longer with up to a dozen episodes a day. The acute diarrhea leads to anemia and renal failure. In some individuals, neurologic problems can result from a severe E. coli enteric infection.

Enteric infections with Staphylococcus aureus produce symptoms of nausea, vomiting, abdominal cramping, and diarrhea within two to eight hours after ingestion of contaminated foods. Fever is not a frequent sign with a Staphylococcus aureus infection. Custard-filled pastries and processed meats are common sources of these enterotoxins.

Clostridium perfringens infection is another food-related infection. The enterotoxins produce symptoms similar to Staphylococcus aureas with diarrhea, abdominal cramps, and occasionally vomiting. The most common source of contamination is food from steam tables that is kept warmed for extended periods of time.

In a common form of infectious gastroenteritis, the bowel wall is invaded by the Salmonella species. This type of infection has another contaminated food connection. Watery diarrhea, cramps, nausea, vomiting, and fever are the signs of Salmonella food poisoning. While it is often a self-limiting illness, debilitated persons are at risk for bacteremia. Although the diarrhea may continue for up to two weeks, the acute symptoms usually appear in 12 to 36 hours and last about five days.

Shigella is transmitted through the fecal-oral route. It symptoms are similar to other enteric infections with the addition of bloody diarrhea, fever, tenesmus, and the laboratory finding of polymorphonuclear leukocytes on diagnostic smears. The sites most often associated with Shigella infection are places where large numbers of people congregate in small spaces with minimal opportunity for hand washing over long periods of time.

Campylobacter jejuni causes more enteric infections in the United States than either Salmonella or Shigella. This organism originates from animals used for nutrition or as pets. Symptoms are consistent with other enteric infections but can last longer and a relapse is possible.

Yersinia enterocolitica causes another self-limiting colitis with fever, right lower quadrant abdominal pain, and diarrhea. This bacterium has been associated with stimulating the onset of Crohn's disease. Arthralgias, polyarthritis, and skin lesions can also result from this organism.

Enteric infections with Vibrio parahaemolyticus can result from eating raw seafood, particularly oysters and sushi-style red snapper and salmon. While self-limiting in nature, this infection causes diarrhea, fever, nausea, vomiting, and abdominal cramping.

When Listeria monocytogenes is present in tainted processed meats and poultry products or in unpasteurized milk products, fever, cramps, myalgias, diarrhea, and headache result. Older adults and immunocompromised persons are at highest risk, with mortality rates of 20 to 30% in the United States.

Contaminated water is the most frequent source of Vibrio cholerae infection. This secretory diarrheal disease is most often identified with the subcontinent of India, Southeast Asia, Africa, and the Middle East. Serious symptoms that often follow the onset are dehydration with volume depletion and metabolic acidosis. If not treated immediately, death may result.

Entamoeba histolytica is a protozoan parasite infection of the GI tract. It is the pathogen that is responsible for the majority of diarrhea in the United States. This is still a small amount of infectious gastroenteritis at approximately 4%. Worldwide, this microorganism infects 50,000,000 people and kills more than 50,000 people yearly (Stanley & Reed, 2001). While most people infected are carriers and do not have symptoms, the causative amoeba can enter the colon wall and result in bloody diarrhea. Infected people are often travelers, tourists, and immigrants from developing countries. It can be spread by anal sexual contact as well.

Cryptosporidium parvum is found in contaminated water. The person ingests oocysts and frequently remains asymptomatic unless they are frail or are immunocompromised. The most common symptoms are profuse watery diarrhea with fever, anorexia, nausea, and vomiting. This can last from one to two weeks. Cryptosporidium parvum is a parasite identified in 400,000 cases in Milwaukee, Wisconsin in 1993 due to the contamination of the municipal water system (Eckmann, & Gillin, 2001; Nasser, Hasan, & Gregg, 2000; Nichols, 1999).

Giardia lamblia is the leading cause of parasitic waterborne diarrhea around the world. This protozoa is found where human sewage and water supplies are mixed. However, this parasite is endemic in some areas of the world (Eckmann, & Gillin, 2001; Richter, 2000).

While the causes of infectious gastroenteritis leading to diarrhea are varied, the most important treatment issue is the rehydration of the patient while the cause is sought. Due to the self-limiting feature of these symptoms, the diarrhea often subsides by the time treatment is sought. Nevertheless, diarrhea can have different outcomes according to the unique situation of the patient. The more vulnerable the patient is to rapid changes in health status, the more aggressive the treatment should be, with rehydration being the key to preventing serious complications.

GENERAL NURSING CARE

Infectious gastroenteritis can be mild and self-limiting, or severe and in need of immediate intervention. The initial inventory of the signs and symptoms along with duration, severity, and other information related to food and fluid sources, contact with potentially infected persons, and recent travel activities are important elements in the patient's history. Categorizing the type of diarrhea as acute, persistent, or chronic is helpful in selecting the protocol that is best for the specific needs of the patient. Identifying distressing symptoms, which are those that force a change in activities such as fever or dysentery, is vital for planning care and identifying differential diagnoses. Oral fluid hydration should be initiated to manage a mild, uncomplicated episode. The recommended fluid is a hypoosmolar solution containing glucose and electrolytes. Two recipes that can be made at home for significant monetary savings while providing essential elements for rehydration are listed in Table 6.2.

ASSESSMENT

Obtaining a thorough history of present illness and exposure to infected persons, food or fluid sources that may be suspect, and a food history that will identify the incubation period of the cause of the illness is essential. Note symptoms of thirst, lassitude, dry mucosa, and decreased skin turgor (avoiding the hands in frail elderly due to their lack of subcutaneous tissue). More severe symptoms can include postural hypotension, delirium, oliguria, and shock (Nichols, 1999). Assess the knowledge level of proper hygiene measures when buying and preparing food, selecting food in eating establishments, and following toileting activities.

PLANNING

Patient education is imperative to prevent disease in the future. Hand washing after toileting, especially after a bowel movement, must be stressed. This will also prevent the spread of the illness to family, friends, coworkers, or acquaintances. Encourage regular drinking of adequate amounts of fluids to reverse and/or avoid dehydration. Instruct in avoiding foods that will aggravate the symptoms, such as caffeine, dairy products, high-fat or high-fiber foods, carbonated beverages, sugar-free products containing Sorbitol, and alcohol (Nichols, 1999).

TABLE 6.2   Rehydrating Solution & Stool Volume Reduction Recipes

Rehydrating Solution (A then B)	Stool Volume Reduction
A. 8 ounces juice (apple or orange) $1/2$ tsp. corn syrup or honey Pinch of salt (stir & drink) B. $1/4$ tsp. baking soda 8 ounce glass of water (stir & drink)	4 cups water $1 1/2$ cups of rice cereal $1/2$ tsp. salt (stir & drink)

Adapted from Nichols, C. H. (1999). Diarrhea. In T. M. Buttaro, J. Trybulski, P. P. Bailey, & J. Sandberg-Cook (Eds.), *Primary care: A collaborative practice.* St. Louis: Mosby.

Planning must include illness prevention measures that include 1) avoiding high-risk foods like raw seafood, raw eggs, unpasteurized dairy products, and undercooked beef and poultry, and 2) avoiding foods that have been left on steam tables for hours, in an outdoor environment without temperature control, or in all-day picnics or food stands. The temperature of food fluctuates dramatically if no temperature control mechanism is in place and this fluctuation leads to rapid growth of dangerous bacteria in food.

Measures that can be effective in reducing the incidence of C. difficile infections and cross-infection include rapid and accurate diagnosis with correct pharmacotherapy if indicated. Most patients with C. difficile infections have recently received antimicrobial therapy—usually clindamycin, cephalosporins, or the extended-spectrum penicillins. The illness is best prevented by limiting the use of broad-spectrum antibiotics (Moyenuddin, Williamson, & Ohl, 2002).

Implementation of enteric precautions for symptomatic patients, reinforcing hand washing, and using daily disinfection in the surrounding environments as well as the immediate environment of the person with C. difficile infection must be included in the immediate plans for patient care and protection from illness transmission (Barbut & Petit, 2001).

NURSING DIAGNOSES AND PLAN OF CARE

1. Knowledge deficit related to causative/contributing factors and therapeutic needs
   Definition: passage of loose, unformed bowel movements (feces)
   Plan of Care: assess causative factors; maintain fluid and electrolyte balance; maintain skin integrity; reestablish and maintain normal pattern of bowel functioning; instruct the patient in the causative factors and rationale for treatment plan.
2. Fluid volume deficit related to excessive losses through the GI tract
   Definition: loss of body fluids from excessive passage of fluid with bowel movements
   Plan of Care: assess causative factors; maintain fluid and electrolyte balance; instruct the patient in the causative factors and rationale for treatment plan.
3. Pain, acute related to abdominal cramping with rapid passage of feces through the GI tract
   Definition: subjective experience of abdominal cramping type pain.

Plan of Care: assess pain using a scale (none = 1; worst = 10); assess causative factors; implement pain relief protocol; evaluate effectiveness of pain relief.

4. Pain, acute related to irritation/excoriation of skin in the anal/perineum area associated with acid content of liquid stool

   Definition: subjective perception of pain with objective assessment of skin condition.

   Plan of Care: assess pain using a scale (none = 1; worst= 10); assess skin integrity; implement skin care protocol (prompt skin cleansing & pericare after each bowel movement, use skin barrier/ointment as needed, dry and clean linens, skin evaluation record); evaluate intervention and skin condition.

5. Skin integrity, impaired, related to effects of liquid, frequent, fecal excretions on sensitive tissue in the anal/perineum area

   Definition: subjective perception of pain with objective assessment of skin condition.

   Plan of Care: assess pain using a scale (none = 1; worst= 10); assess skin integrity; implement skin care protocol (prompt skin cleansing & pericare after each bowel movement, use skin barrier/ointment as needed, dry and clean linens, skin evaluation record); evaluate intervention and skin condition (Doegnes, Moorhouse, & Geissler-Murr, 2002).

INTERVENTIONS, TREATMENTS, ALTERNATIVE TREATMENTS

Hydration. Improving or maintaining hydration during the acute symptoms while waiting for resolution of the underlying cause will support the majority of symptomatic patients. Carbonated beverages that have been allowed to remain open to the air causing the loss of the carbonation can be taken as water substitutes. When oral fluids can't be taken in sufficient quantities to maintain normal hydration, intravenous solutions may be needed. This will require a trip to a health care facility to determine the accurate fluid needs and treatment. Electrolytes that are lost with diarrhea and often need replacement are sodium, potassium, bicarbonate, and chlorine (Richter, 2000).

Nutrition. As symptoms begin to resolve and stools become more formed, solid foods can be added to the diet. If bloating occurs with the addition of dairy products, withdraw them for one to two days and then reintroduce them again. Bloating is a sign of lactose intolerance after the bowel has begun to return to normal. If bloating returns after a nondairy waiting period, suspect other causes for the diarrhea or irritable bowel syndrome (Porth, 1998). See chapter 10, Irritable Bowel Syndrome, for additional information.

Pharmacotherapy. The treatment of symptoms using medications is often dependent upon the stool culture results. Not all bacteria are treated with the same or similar pharmacotherapeutic agents. When the cause is parasitic in origin, definitive antimicrobial drugs are appropriate. The following discussion of drug therapy addresses the different causes and needs when infectious diarrhea is the predominant symptom.

Antimotility drugs should be avoided in cases of infectious gastroenteritis. Preventing the expulsion of the pathogen may prove more harmful than the increased motility of the bowel in diarrhea. Noninflammatory diarrhea responds well to antimotility drugs such as loperamide (Immodium), two 2 mg tablets at onset, then one 2 mg tablet after each loose stool, not to exceed 16 mg in a single 24-hour period. Diphenoxylate (Lomotil), taken as two (2.5 or 5 mg) tablets every four to six hours, up to 20 mg daily. Tincture of opium (0.5 to 1 mL) five to ten drops every four to six hours, and paregoric 4 mL every four hours, as well as codeine (30 to 60 mg) every four hours are effective treatments of diarrhea by inhibition of intestinal motility. If Shigella is the causative organism, these drugs should not be used. An infection with E. coli O157:H7 also should not be treated with antimotility drugs.

Nausea is commonly treated with promethazine (Phenergan), or prochlorperazine (Compazine).The symptom of vomiting is usually seen in viral caused gastroenteritis, associated with contaminated food or water, and treatment is aimed at alleviating the vomiting and abdominal cramping. These symptoms are self-limiting and prevention of dehydration and electrolyte imbalance is the goal.

Absorbent medications. Abdominal cramping responds to absorbents. An example of this is kaolin-pectin preparations (Kaopectate) and Donnatal. Four tablespoons of kaolin-pectin is given every four hours for reduction of cramping. Donnatal, one or two tablets, is given three times daily for relief of cramping. The use of bismuth subsalicylate (Pepto-Bismol) must be used cautiously in older adults with comorbidities. If anticoagulation drugs such as Warfarin are taken, bismuth can affect the anticoagulation process. Immunocompromised persons should avoid bismuth or bismuth preparations due to the possibility of encephalopathy (Nichols, 1999).

Antibiotics. Older adults suspected of Salmonella bacteremia who have vascular prostheses (e.g., heart valve) should receive prophylactic antibiotics to prevent generalized sepsis.

The first drug of choice in the treatment for Clostridium difficile is metronidazole. Oral vancomycin is usually reserved for persons who can't tolerate oral metronidazole or do not respond to that drug. Metronidazole is absorbed from the upper GI tract and may cause side effects. Vancomycin is poorly absorbed, and its actions are limited to the GI tract (Porth, 1998).

The use of antibiotics is not recommended routinely for acute bacterial diarrheas because most infections are self-limited. Shigellosis is one of the few bacterium caused diarrhea that responds to antibiotics. Oral amoxicillin, 500 mg three times daily for three to five days, is commonly prescribed for Shigellosis (Oldfield & Wallace, 2001; Richter, 2000).

Illness brought about by Campylobacter can be treated with erythromycin, 500 mg four times daily for one full week. Likewise, severe or toxic Yersinia infection is treated with chloramphenicol, 50 mg per kilogram of weight, four times daily for one full week (Richter, 2000).

The danger of inducing diarrhea with the use of antibiotics is the risk that makes empirical treatment unattractive. Antibiotic resistance must be considered before using these drugs (Richter, 2000). However, some clinicians prefer empirical treatment with Ciprofloxacin, 500 mg twice daily for three days, or with norfloxacin, 400 mg twice a day for three days, while waiting for the stool cultures to return from the laboratory. If Giardia is the causative agent and the diarrhea continues for two weeks, metronidazole (Flagyl), 250 mg four times a day for one week, or quinacrine, 100 mg three times a day for one week, can be prescribed (Oldfield & Wallace, 2001; Richter, 2000).

HEALTH PROMOTION AND QUALITY OF LIFE ISSUES

Health promotion is the maintenance of living conditions that support a lifestyle aimed at the highest possible state of wellness. This requires active participation in health problem solving situations. Understanding health conditions that may not be optimal, then making rational and informed decisions regarding health care needs, is essential to successful health promotion. Quality of life is enhanced for the older adult when their self-care focuses on maintaining independence with perceived life satisfaction (Pender, Murdaugh, & Parsons, 2002).

The ability to enjoy meals served in restaurants, at friend's homes, at picnics or other public events can provide significant social interaction and enjoyment for older adults. The dangers that can be encountered at these events include food poisoning in mild, moderate, or severe cases.

Infectious gastroenteritis is a frequent health risk at events where the food is not maintained in temperature controlled environments. Awareness of the potential for food-borne illnesses is essential for health promotion and illness prevention strategies.

Other health-promoting and health-protecting behaviors include food preparation in the home. Proper cleaning of food preparation surfaces and cooking utensils is the foundation for safe cooking. Cleaning and cooking meat, poultry, fish, pork, and other protein sources at recommended temperatures to eliminate the source of food-borne illnesses should be stressed in each teaching session.

Hand washing is imperative to prevent the transmission of bacteria, viruses, and parasites. The use of sufficient soap to lather the hands followed by rinsing under running water until all of the soap is gone may need to be reinforced at every opportunity. Signage in health care facilities, restaurants, and public restrooms is a tool used to reinforce hand washing. Eliminating the fecal-oral route of infection transmission should be a primary aim of public health education.

FOLLOW-UP CARE

When bacterial infectious gastroenteritis is reported to the health department in a city, town, village, or county within the United States, a health care worker is sent to interview and obtain a stool culture for examination. If the epidemiology of the infection leads to a restaurant or other public place where food is served, an investigation will be made at that facility. Licensing and grading of the establishment can be adversely affected if a cause of infectious gastroenteritis is found.

The individual with the infection will need to have specimen collections and cultures done by a public health care worker for several months following the diagnosis. If the infected individual is employed in a sensitive setting such as working around food, sick persons, or providing physical care to others, employment may be suspended until negative cultures are obtained over time in order to prevent spreading the infection.

CONCLUSION

Infectious gastroenteritis is caused by a variety of organisms that may have an extremely varied presentation, course, and treatment response. The data presented in this chapter provide insights into the pathophysiology of these various organisms and their clinical presentation. As a better understanding of the colon and its immunologic defense mechanisms becomes better known by health care professionals, identification and treatment options for the various organisms will most likely produce better results in controlling the symptoms. The pathophysiological understanding of this illness will hopefully reduce the amount of antibiotics used inappropriately to treat infectious diarrhea. The cost of antibiotics and the potential to worsen the already significant problem of antibiotic resistance of enteric pathogens must be considered prior to the empirical treatment of diarrhea with these agents. Only the prudent use of antimicrobials is indicated for infectious gastroenteritis.

REFERENCES

Barbut, F., & Petit, J. C. (2001). Epidemiology of Clostridium difficile-associated infections. *Clinical Microbial Infection, 8,* 405–410.

Doenges, M. E., Moorhouse, M. F., & Geissler-Murr, A. C. (2002). *Nurse's pocket guide: Diagnoses, interventions, and rationales,* 8 ed. Philadelphia: F. A. Davis Company.

Eckmann, L., & Gillin, F. D. (2001). Microbes and microbial toxins: Paradigms for microbial-mucosal interactions, Part I. Pathophysiological aspects of enteric infections with the lumen-dwelling protozoan pathogen Giardia lamblia. *American Journal of Physiology—Gastrointestinal and Liver Physiology, 280*(1), G1–G6.

Moyenuddin, M., Williamson, J. C., & Ohl, C. A. (2002). Clostridium difficile-associated diarrhea: Current strategies for diagnosis and therapy. *Current Gastroenterology Reports, 4,* 279–286.

Nassar, N. N., Hasan, M. S., & Gregg, C. R. (2000). Infectious diarrhea. In L. E. Bilhartz & C. L. Croft, *Gastrointestinal disease in primary care.* Philadelphia: Lippincott Williams & Wilkins.

National Center for Infectious Diseases (2001). *Viral gastroenteritis.* Atlanta, GA: Center for Disease Control and Prevention.

Nichols, C. H. (1999). Diarrhea. In T. M. Buttaro, J. Trybulski, P. P. Bailey, & J. Sandberg-Cook (Eds.), *Primary care: A collaborative practice.* St. Louis: Mosby.

Oldfield, E. C. 3rd, & Wallace, M. R. (2001). The role of antibiotics in the treatment of infectious diarrhea. *Gastroenterology Clinics of North America,* Sep. 30(3), 817–836.

Pender, N. J., Murdaugh, C. L., & Parsons, M. A. (2002). *Health promotion in nursing practice,* 4 ed. Upper Saddle River, NJ: Prentice Hall.

Porth, C. M. (1998). *Pathophysiology: Concepts of altered health states,* 5 ed. Philadelphia: Lippincott Publishing.

Richter, J. M. (2000). Evaluation and management of diarrhea. In A. H. Goroll & A. G. Mulley, Jr., 4 ed. *Primary care medicine: Office evaluation and management of the adult patient.* Philadelphia: Lippincott, Williams & Wilkins.

Stanley, S. L., & Reed, S. L. (2001). Microbes and microbial toxins: Paradigms for microbial-mucosal interactions Part 6, Entamoeba histolytica: Parasite-host interactions. *American Journal of Physiology—Gastrointestinal and Liver Physiology, 280*(1), G1049–G1054.

$-7-$

Vitamin B$_{12}$ and Folate Deficiencies

Lori Candela

Vitamin deficiencies are relatively common among the elderly. Nearly one-third of all older individuals have been shown to have vitamin or trace element deficiencies (Gary & Fluery, 2002). A decrease in energy intake and overall diet quality has been associated with increasing age. However, dietary vitamin requirements are often the same or even higher as for younger age groups. Vitamin B$_{12}$ and folate are among the long list of vitamins and minerals requiring gastrointestinal digestion and absorption in order to be utilized by the body. A deficiency in either can result in a wide variety of potentially deadly symptoms. Despite this, relatively little information is available regarding how the aging process specifically affects digestion, absorption, and use of vitamins by the body.

Vitamin B$_{12}$ deficiency is a common occurrence in the elderly, with an incidence rate as high as 15% (Groff & Gropper, 2000). The incidence was even higher in the Framingham Heart Study, in which 18% of 22–63-year-olds had decreased vitamin B$_{12}$ levels compared with 40% in the 65–99 age group (Brown, 2002). The extent of the problem in the elderly population is even more significant as 15% of those over the age of 60 have undiagnosed vitamin B$_{12}$ deficiency (Andres, Kurtz, Perrin, Maloisel, Demangeat, Goichot, et al., 2001).

Vitamin B$_{12}$ (cobalamin), the last of the vitamins to be identified, is now known to affect metabolic processes that are essential to the normal

81

functioning of all cells, particularly cells of the nervous system, bone marrow, and gastrointestinal tract. Folate (folic acid) also affects cell metabolism, particularly in red and white blood cell formation and maturation.

Vitamin B_{12} and folate are interrelated in many ways. Both are required for normal body functioning and must come from foods in the diet, dietary supplements, or parental forms. In order to be properly absorbed, vitamin B_{12} and folate require an intact gastrointestinal tract. Both are also important in homocysteine metabolism. Folic acid is broken down through enzymatic reduction to become 5-methyltetrahydrofolate. This substrate functions as a methyl donor in a complex remethylation process in which homocysteine is synthesized to form methionine. Vitamin B_{12} shares an important role as well, serving as a cofactor in the synthesis of methionine. A deficiency in either vitamin B_{12} or folate can result in impaired conversion of homocysteine to methionine, resulting in increased plasma homocysteine levels (Gerhard & Duell, 1999). Elevated homocysteine levels have been implicated in the development of atherosclerotic disease and coronary artery disease. Both vitamin B_{12} and folate deficiencies result in anemia, often with abnormally large (megaloblastic) red blood cells noted upon examination of the mean cell volume (MCV) of the red blood cell indices (Mahan & Escott-Stump, 2000).

Low folate stores are noted in 10% of the general population (Mahan & Escott-Stump, 2000). In the elderly, folate deficiency may be one of the most common causes of nutritional deficiency, affecting 3–7% of elderly persons (McCool, Huls, Peppones, & Schlenker, 2001; Shils, Olson, Shike, & Ross, 1999). While the presence of atrophic gastritis (a common gastrointestinal disorder in the elderly) decreases absorption of folate, this is somewhat countered by bacterial overgrowth, which tends to synthesize folate (Shils, Olson, Shike, & Ross, 1999).

Like so many disorders in the elderly, the presentation of vitamin B_{12} or folate deficiency may not be clear. The usual sign of pallor is more difficult to assess in the elderly. Other signs such as weakness, fatigue, and shortness of breath are vague, and many elderly tend to see these signs as a normal part of aging. Often, the first sign is a worsening of a preexisting condition, such as congestive heart failure, or neurological deterioration, i.e., apathy, dizziness, or cognitive impairment (Smith, 2000).

The treatment goal is centered on the achievement of adequate body requirements of vitamin B_{12} and folate. The plan of action for an elderly person with vitamin B_{12} or folate deficiency must include attention to sensory or perceptual alterations, increased risk for injury, and potential ineffective management of the therapeutic regimen. See Table 7.1.

TABLE 7.1   Definitions Associated With Vitamin B$_{12}$ and Folate

Achlorhydria:	absence of hydrochloric acid
Adenosylcobalamin:	one of two active cofactor forms of vitamin B$_{12}$
Cobalamin:	chemical name for vitamin B$_{12}$
Cyancobalamin:	name used interchangeably with cobalamin in the literature to describe vitamin B$_{12}$
Folic acid:	the synthetic form of folate
Homocysteine:	a sulfhydryl-containing amino acid derived from the metabolism of dietary methionine
Hypochlorhydria:	deficiency of gastric hydrochloric acid
Intrinsic factor:	protein secreted by the gastric parietal cells
Methionine:	an essential amino acid, abundant in animal sources of protein
Methylcobalamin:	one of two active cofactor forms of vitamin B$_{12}$
Methylmalonic acid:	metabolite normally found in small amounts in the body; levels rise in vitamin B$_{12}$ deficiency, but not in folate deficiency
Schilling test:	diagnostic test to determine cobalamin absorption deficiencies
R factor:	competes with intrinsic factor to bind with intestinal vitamin B$_{12}$; vitamin B$_{12}$ bound to R factor cannot be absorbed
R protein:	carrier glycoprotein for vitamin B$_{12}$, found in saliva, bile, gastric and intestinal juice, and serum
Transcobalamin (TC):	TC I and TC II carrier proteins for vitamin B$_{12}$ in the plasma

ETIOLOGY

A deficiency in either vitamin B$_{12}$ or folate may be due to inadequate dietary intake, malnutrition, chronic, significant alcohol intake, problems with gastrointestinal absorption, history of gastric surgery, severe Crohn's disease, pancreatic insufficiency, or the use of certain drugs. Additionally, a vitamin B$_{12}$ deficiency may be related to the absence of intrinsic factor (pernicious anemia), transcobalamin II deficiency, or more rarely, intestinal parasites.

Vitamin B$_{12}$ is synthesized from bacteria and is found in all animal sources. Strict vegetarians (those who do not consume any animal, fish, or dairy products) are at highest risk for vitamin B$_{12}$ deficiency unless their diet is supplemented with vitamins (Mahan & Escott-Stump, 2000). With the exception of strict vegetarians, vitamin B$_{12}$ deficiency due to low dietary intake is rare; though it is seen more commonly among the elderly in institutions (Schils, Olson, Shike, & Ross, 1999). The recommended daily intake (RDI) of vitamin B$_{12}$ is 2.4 micrograms per day for males and females over the age of 51. However, the actual intake for the elderly population is generally much higher, 7.1 micrograms and 7.4 micrograms for males and females, respectively (Brown, 2000). Despite adequate consumption, the elderly are more prone to vitamin deficiencies due to decreased absorption. Atrophic gastritis, alcohol use, gastrointestinal disorders, particularly of the jejunum, and certain medications commonly used by the elderly, such as antacids, diuretics, and anti-inflammatory drugs all contribute to decreased vitamin absorption (Brown, 2002). About 50% of the vitamin B_{12} in the body is stored in the liver (Shils, Olson, Shike, & Ross, 1999). Since total body content of vitamin B_{12} (including what is stored in the liver) is around 3–5 milligrams and daily losses are usually only 3–5 micrograms per day, it could take more than three years to see any deficiency (Tierny, McPhee, & Papadakis, 2000).

The RDI for folate is 400 micrograms per day. Unlike vitamin B_{12}, most elderly do not meet daily requirements for folate intake. Folate is found in animal and plant sources, however, some 50–90% of folate is lost during storage and cooking of foods (Mahan & Escott-Stump, 2000). The body stores of folate are small, compared with vitamin B_{12}, generally 2–3 months' worth; thus deficiency may develop much more quickly (Snow, 1999; Tierney, McPhee, & Papadakis, 2000).

PATHOLOGY

Generally, vitamin B_{12} and folate are bound to food proteins. Absorption requires that vitamin B_{12} and folate be split from these proteins, which requires the presence of gastric acid and pepsin. These gastric acids may be severely diminished in people with chronic atrophic gastritis, which may affect as many as 30% of the elderly (Brown, 2002). The condition leads to thinning and degeneration of the stomach wall. Degeneration of the gastric mucosa results in gastric cell atrophy and decreased secretion of stomach acids (Huether & McCance, 2000).

Helicobacter pylori is frequently associated with atrophic gastritis, which leads to gastric inflammation and a further decrease in gastric acid production (Brown, 2002). The organism is very prevalent; in fact, it is among the most common causes of gastric infections in the world. Nearly one half of adults harbor the organism in developed countries and some 90% in developing countries. It is a very common cause of peptic ulcer disease and chronic superficial gastritis, which leads to gastric gland atrophy. The relationship of *Helicobacter pylori* as a cause of vitamin B_{12} deficiency has been examined. In a study of 138 patients with anemia and vitamin B_{12}

deficiency, the eradication of *Helicobacter pylori* alone improved anemia status and low vitamin levels in 40% of those infected with the bacteria (Kaptan, Beyan, Ural, Cetin, Avcu, Gulsen, et al., 2000).

While abdominal surgery can impair the absorption of many nutrients needed by the body, the inability of the body to absorb vitamin B$_{12}$ and folate can lead to nutritional deficiencies. Specifically, the surgical procedures known as gastrectomy, or partial gastrectomy may impair vitamin B$_{12}$ absorption, while jejunal surgery is more likely to decrease folate absorption (Mahan & Escott-Stump, 2000). Following total gastrectomy, there is a loss of intrinsic factor secreting cells, hydrochloric acid, and pepsin-secreting cells, eventually resulting in an inability to absorb vitamin B$_{12}$. While partial gastrectomy does not directly cause decreased vitamin B$_{12}$ absorption, eventually atrophic gastritis develops, ultimately resulting in decreased vitamin absorption. Another gastrointestinal operation frequently resulting in vitamin B$_{12}$ deficiency is Billroth II surgery. Following surgery, patients develop gastric bacterial overgrowth. Bacterial uptake of vitamin B$_{12}$ limits the total amount available for gastrointestinal absorption. As previously noted, small bowel bacteria tend to produce folate, thus increasing rather than deceasing the amount available for absorption (McNally, 2001).

After being freed from food proteins, vitamin B$_{12}$ is picked up by R proteins and carried toward the ileum. Pancreatic enzymes are necessary to split the R proteins away from the vitamin in order for it to bind with intrinsic factor. Folate absorption requires these digestive enzymes in order to hydrolyze the ingested vitamin into a form easily absorbed in the jejunum. Therefore, any pancreatic insufficiency can lead to decreased vitamin B$_{12}$ or folate absorption due to reduced pancreatic enzymes (Mahan & Escott-Stump, 2000; Shils, Olson, Shike, & Ross, 1999).

Several medications impede the absorption of vitamin B$_{12}$ and folate. "Medications commonly used by older adults, such as antacids, diuretics, phenytoin (Dilantin), sulfonamides, and anti-inflammatory drugs affect folate metabolism" (Brown, 2002, p. 438). Vitamin B$_{12}$ absorption is impaired by medications such as colchicines, neomycin, omeprazole, and p-aminosallicylic acid (Snow, 1999).

Crohn's disease has been associated with multiple vitamin deficiencies. Although it can occur anywhere throughout the gastrointestinal system, the ileum is a common site. Severe vitamin malabsorption is due to ongoing bowel inflammation and/or surgical resection (Kastin & Buchman, 2002).

Pernicious anemia is an absolute deficiency of intrinsic factor, which prevents vitamin B$_{12}$ from being absorbed, although a small amount of the vitamin may still be absorbed through passive diffusion. Under normal conditions, once vitamin B_{12} has been split from carrier food proteins, it is able to bind with intrinsic factor. The vitamin B_{12}/intrinsic factor complex is taken up by receptors in the terminal ileum for transport across membranes and into the circulation.

The lack of intrinsic factor may be congenital or acquired, as with atrophic gastritis. Nearly 90% of those with pernicious anemia have serum autoantibodies to gastric parietal cells or to intrinsic factor itself. Interestingly, the percentage of those with parietal cell autoantibodies increases with age; rising from 2.5% in the third decade to 9.6% in the eighth decade (Baik & Russell, 1999).

Occasionally, intestinal parasites, such as the broad fish tapeworm (*Diphyllobothrium latum*) may be identified as the source for vitamin B_{12} deficiency. The parasites are ingested in raw or undercooked fish, often pike or salmon, and attach to the wall of the small intestine. Vitamin B_{12} absorption becomes impaired due to uptake of the vitamin by the worms (Tierney, McPhee, & Papadakis, 2000).

Once taken up by receptors in the terminal ileum, vitamin B_{12} is released from the intrinsic factor and binds to transcobalamin proteins for transport through the circulation. Congenital transcobalamin II deficiency is an autosomal recessive disorder. The cause is unclear but may relate to defects in the intrinsic factor vitamin B_{12} receptor or in postreceptor pathways. In infancy, this disorder is manifested by the presence of megaloblastic anemia and normal vitamin levels. Treatment includes massive vitamin doses. This is done in order to facilitate passive diffusion of the vitamin, which occurs normally at a fraction of rate of active transcobalamin transport (McNally, 2001; Snow, 1999).

RELATIONSHIP TO HOMOCYSTEINE

Serum homocysteine levels may rise in the presence of either a vitamin B_{12} or folate deficiency. Elevated homocysteine levels have been associated with increased risk for cardiovascular disease in cross sectional and retrospective studies, though this risk is not well established in prospective studies (Hankey & Eikelboom, 2001). However, the link between high homocysteine levels and arterial vascular disease is established. The mechanism is not entirely clear, but may involve injury and changes to vessel walls (Gemmati, Previati, Serino, Moratelli, Guerra, Capitani, et al., 1999). Vitamins B_6 and B_{12} and folate share common metabolic pathways with homocysteine. Deficiencies in any of these three can result in increased synthesis of homocysteine. "After confirmation of high homocysteine concentration, it is important to check the vitamin status owing to the inverse relationships reported between homocysteine and blood levels of folate, concentrations with plasma/serum levels of folic acid, vitamin B$_{12}$, and vitamin B$_6$" (Malinow, Bostom, & Krauss, 1999, p. 181).

VITAMIN DEFICIENCY AND CELLULAR FUNCTION

The signs and symptoms of vitamin B$_{12}$ or folate deficiency relate to alterations in cellular development and function. The impaired biosynthesis of DNA and RNA results in decreases in cellular division. This is especially noticeable in rapidly dividing cells, such red and white blood cells, epithelial cells, and some neurological cells (Mahon & Escott-Stump, 2000). The severity of anemia is variable; hematocrits may fall to 10–15%, with associated increases in fatigue and general weakness. The mean cell volume (MCV) may be increased or may be normal. The changes in mucosal cells can lead to a variety of gastrointestinal symptoms, such as anorexia or diarrhea (Tierney, McPhee, & Papadakis, 2000).

VITAMIN DEFICIENCY AND NEUROLOGICAL EFFECTS

Vitamin B$_{12}$ deficiency can lead to neurological deficits, which, if untreated, may be irreversible (Snow, 1999). Chronically low levels lead to impaired myelin synthesis. Eventually, demyelination occurs in the nerve tracts and axons (Shils, Olson, Shike, & Ross, 1999; Browning, 2002). Both vitamin B$_{12}$ and folate have important roles in properly functioning metabolic brain pathways. Low vitamin levels lead to hypomethylation, which, as previously noted, reduces the synthesis of methionine. It also decreases the synthesis of S-adenosylmethionine (SAMe), which is an important methyl donor in many CNS reactions. Hypomethylation results in the inhibition of methylation reactions involving membrane phospholipids, proteins, and neurotransmitter metabolism such as dopamine, serotonin, and norepinephrine. Other neurocognitive changes may result from the chronically high homocysteine levels associated with vitamin B$_{12}$ and folate deficiency that result in arterial vascular damage (Calvaresi & Bryan, 2001).

The variety of neurological symptoms may include peripheral nerve parasthesias (particularly in the hands and feet), a sense of clumsiness, balance difficulties, vision complaints (such as loss of central vision or acquired yellow/blue color blindness), confusion, memory loss, poor judgment, dementia, or even severe paranoia, sometimes referred to as "megaloblastic madness" (Browning, 2002). Generally, if neurological symptoms have been present for less than six months, treatment may reverse impairments (Tierney, McPhee, & Papadakis, 2000).

GENERAL NURSING CARE

The vague symptoms, along with lack of consistency in blood cell indices, make history taking and proper diagnostic testing essential. It is important to assess for any history of gastrointestinal disease or intestinal surgery that may affect absorption (Brown, 2002). Nutrition history and use of any over the counter supplements as well as prescribed medications is also very important.

Diagnostic tests may include serum vitamin levels and red blood cell folate levels. If the levels are normal but the symptoms strongly suggest a deficiency, serum homocysteine and methyl malonic acid levels may need to be examined. Additionally, a Schilling test may be performed if vitamin malabsorption is suspected (Browning, 2002). However, the need to perform a Schilling test has recently been called into question. Studies have been conducted in which high doses of oral vitamin have treated all types of deficiency. Thus there is less need for the additional time and cost of obtaining a Schilling test (Smith, 2000).

The often vague and insidious presentation of the elderly person with vitamin B_{12} or folate deficiency is a challenge. Often the patient is not anemic. Cobalamin levels and mean cell volume (MCV) may be normal. Because of the vague nature of the symptoms, some experts have begun to call for periodic vitamin B_{12} deficiency screening in those over the age of 51, which would include serum levels of methyl malonic acid and/or homocysteine (Kapadia, 2000).

NURSING DIAGNOSIS AND PLAN OF CARE

Altered nutrition: less than body requirements for vitamin B_{12} and/or folate related to:

1. decreased oral intake of foods high in vitamin and/or folate associated with

    a. anorexia, diminished sense of smell/taste, early satiety
    b. difficulty chewing and swallowing associated with poor dentition
    c. difficulty with purchasing and/or preparing healthy foods
2. reduced absorption of nutrients related to:
    a. hypochlorhydria, decreased intestinal blood flow, atrophy of intestinal cells
    b. gastric or intestinal surgery
    c. intestinal disorders, i.e., Crohn's disease
    d. medications interfering with intestinal absorption

Outcome: patient will maintain adequate vitamin nutrition as evidenced by:
    a. hematocrit, hemoglobin, red blood cell count, leukocyte count, mean cell volume within normal limits for patient
    b. usual strength and activity tolerance
    c. able to obtain and prepare foods high in vitamin B$_{12}$ and folate content

INTERVENTIONS, TREATMENTS, ALTERNATIVE TREATMENTS

Assess for and report signs and symptoms of vitamin B$_{12}$/folate deficiency:

1. low hematocrit, red blood cell count, white cell count, platelet count, low or high mean cell volume
2. fatigue and weakness
3. sore, inflamed mucous membranes
4. pale conjunctiva
5. yellowish tint to skin

Monitor percentage and type of food intake

Implement measures to maintain adequate vitamin B$_{12}$ intake:

1. discuss current dietary practices
2. obtain dietary and/or social service consult if necessary to assist in decreasing barriers to obtaining healthy foods and teaching regarding selecting and preparing foods
3. encourage rest periods before meals if patient suffers from fatigue
4. assure oral care prior to meals and that dentures are inserted properly
5. obtain dental consult if dentures do not fit properly
6. serve small, frequent meals

Implement measures to compensate for taste/smell alterations and dislike of diet

1. serve foods warm to stimulate sense of smell
2. instruct on use of seasonings and flavorings, such as herbs and sweeteners, unless contraindicated
3. limit fluid intake with meals
4. allow adequate time for meals, even if this means reheating
5. administer supplemental vitamin B_{12}/folate as ordered

Risk for injury (falls) related to weakness and loss of balance associated with vitamin B_{12} deficiency

Outcome: patient will not experience falls

Correct underlying vitamin B_{12}/folate deficiency

1. proper dietary practices
2. oral or parenteral supplementations as ordered

Implement measures to reduce risk of falls

1. keep needed items within easy reach
2. keep bed in low position with rails up
3. instruct patient to wear well-fitting shoes/slippers with nonslip soles and no heels
4. keep floor free of clutter, avoid scatter rugs that do not have nonskid surface
5. encourage slow changes of position (1-2 minutes of rest after each change)
6. provide ambulatory aids (walker, cane) as needed
7. instruct patient to move slowly, use a wider stance when walking, and avoid turning head or body rapidly
8. if vision is impaired, orient patient to surroundings, arrangement of furniture, and any obstacles that may be encountered when walking

Ineffective management of therapeutic regimen related to:

a. knowledge deficit regarding diagnosis, diet, medications, and consequences of not complying with treatment plan
b. lack of motivation or inadequate support systems
c. confusion associated with vitamin deficiency

Outcome: patient will demonstrate the probability of regimen compliance as evidence by:

a. statements reflecting ways to integrate diet and medications into lifestyle

    b. willingness to learn and participate in therapeutic regimen
    c. statements reflecting an understanding of consequences with noncompliance to therapeutic regimen

Assess for indications that patient may be unable to manage therapeutic regimen

1. statements reflecting inability to manage care in home setting
2. failure to adhere to treatment plan
3. statements reflecting a lack of understanding of the factors that will worsen condition
4. statements reflecting an unwillingness or inability to modify dietary habits and integrate treatment regimen into lifestyle
5. statements reflecting view that situation is hopeless and compliance is useless

Implement measures to promote effective management of the therapeutic regimen

1. discuss factors with patient that may interfere with management of care (financial difficulties, religious or cultural conflicts, lack of support systems)
2. assist patient in clarifying values and identify ways to incorporate therapeutic goals into value system
3. encourage questions and clarify any misconceptions regarding diagnosis and treatment plan
4. promote actions to promote trust in caregivers (validate conflicting evidence, explain reasons for treatment plan)
5. encourage patient to participate in treatment plan as fully as possible
6. provide oral and written instructions regarding diet and any medication supplements
7. reinforce behaviors suggesting future compliance with the therapeutic regimen (statements reflecting plans to integrate diet and any oral supplements into lifestyle, active participation in achieving dietary and supplemental compliance) (Ulrich & Canale, 2001).

HEALTH PROMOTION AND QUALITY OF LIFE ISSUES

Examination of the elderly diet may reveal consumption of foods that have little nutritional value. Folate is available in many animal and plant foods including liver, beef, white beans, spinach, broccoli, lettuce, cabbage, and eggs (Mahan & Escott-Stump, 2000). It is important to remember that folates are susceptible to oxidation when heated, resulting in the loss of 50% or more of the folate in the cooked food (Snow, 1999). Foods highest in folate include ready-to-eat fortified cereals, citrus products (i.e., orange and grapefruit juice), and yeast breads. The fortification of grain products with folate began in the 1990s and should increase average daily intake by 70 to 120 mcg (Brown, 2002). See Table 7.2.

HOME MANAGEMENT AND SELF-CARE ISSUES

Cognitive impairment that may accompany vitamin B_{12} deficiency, or the generalized weakness associated with related anemia may certainly affect the ability of the elderly person to care for himself/herself in the home setting. This is particularly true if there are inadequate or absent support systems. Assessment may reveal the need for assistance with shopping or preparation of foods. The patient may require assistance in acquiring the resources to meet these needs, such as a personal care attendant. Community resources may include Meals on Wheels or connecting to local senior centers that serve meals.

FOLLOW-UP CARE

Once supplementation for vitamin B_{12} has begun, patients may quickly notice an improved sense of well being (Tierney, McPhee, & Papadakis, 2000) If megaloblastic anemia is present, reticulocyte counts will increase within 2–3 days, red blood cell count within 1 week (normalizing in 4–8 weeks), and mean cell volume should normalize within 78 days (Snow,

TABLE 7.2   Leading Sources of Vitamin B_{12} and Folate

Vitamin B_{12}	Folate
clams	liver
oysters	dark green leafy vegetables
crab	dried beans
liver	green vegetables
beef	oranges
milk	avocados
kidney	whole-wheat products

1999). Supplementation may be started when serum levels reach to 150–250 pmol/L (Cotter & Strumpf, 2002). If the cause of the disorder is severely decreased or absent intrinsic factor, the person may require intramuscular injections for life, often starting with daily for one week (100 to 1000 micrograms each dose), then weekly for one month, and monthly thereafter (Tierney, McPhee, & Papadakis, 2000; Kastin & Buchman, 2002). For patients who cannot tolerate intramuscular dosing, oral preparations can be used. It will take approximately 1000 micrograms orally to achieve 10 micrograms of absorbed vitamin B$_{12}$ (Kastin & Buchman, 2002). Vitamin B$_{12}$ is also available by intranasal route, although the cost is higher and is recommended to start only after serum levels are restored (Cotter & Strumpf, 2002). The risk for permanent neurological damage is so significant if untreated, regular, periodic screenings for vitamin B$_{12}$ have been recommended by some experts (McCool, Huls, Peppones, & Schlenker, 2001).

Folic acid supplementation ranges from 400–1000 micrograms per day (Cotter & Strumpf, 2002). It is important to remember that folic acid supplementation alone may mask vitamin B$_{12}$ deficiency and allow progressive neurological symptoms to continue (Verhaar, Stroes, & Rabelink, 2002). Because folate levels deplete so quickly, follow-up should continue to be every 3–6 months, once levels are stabilized.

REFERENCES

Andres, E., Kurtz, J. E., Perrin, A. E., Maloisel, F., Demangeat, C., Goichot, B., & Schlienger, J. L. (2001). Oral cobalamin therapy for the treatment of patients with food-cobalamin malabsorption. *The American Journal of Medicine, 111*(2), 126–129.

Baik, H. W., & Russell, R. M. (1999). Vitamin B$_{12}$ deficiency in the elderly. *Annual Review of Nutrition, 19*, 357–378.

Brown, J. E. (2002). *Nutrition through the life cycle* (pp. 422–447, 470–474). Belmont, CA: Wadsworth/Thomson Learning.

Browning, R. H. (2002). What's wrong with this patient. *Registered Nurse, 65*(1), 47–49.

Calvaresi, E., & Bryan, J. (2001). B vitamins, cognition, and aging. *Journal of Gerontology, 56B*(6), 327–339.

Cotter, V. T., & Strumpf, N. E. (2002). *Advanced practice nursing with older adults: Clinical guidelines* (pp. 207–208, 289). New York: McGraw-Hill.

Gary, R., & Fluery, J. (2002). Nutritional status: Key to preventing functional decline in hospitalized older people. *Topics in Geriatric Rehabilitation, 17*(3), 40–52.

Gemmati, D., Previati, M., Serino, M. L., Moratelli, S., Guerra, S., Capitani, S., Forini, E., Ballerini, G., & Scapoli, G. L. (1999). Low folate levels and thermolabile methylenetetrahydrofolate reductase as primary determinate of mild hyperhomocystinemia in normal and thromboembolic subjects. *Arteriosclerosis, Thrombosis, and Vascular Biology, 19*(7), 1761–1767.

Gerhard, G. T., & Duell, P. B. (1999). Homocysteine and atherosclerosis. *Current Opinion in Lipidology, 10*(5), 417–429.

Groff, J. L., & Gropper, S. S. (2000). *Advanced nutrition and human metabolism* (pp. 298–304). Belmont, CA: Wadsworth/Thomson Learning.

Hankey, G. J., & Eikelboom, J. W. (2001). Homocysteine and stroke. *Current Opinion in Neurology, 14*(1), 95–102.

Huether, S. E., & McCance, K. L. (2000). *Understanding pathophysiology* (2nd ed.) (p. 519). St. Louis, MO: Mosby.

Kapadia, C. (2000). Cobalamin (vitamin B_{12}) deficiency: Is it a problem for our aging population and is the problem compounded by drugs that inhibit gastric acid secretion. *Journal of Clinical Gastroenterology, 30*(1), 4–6.

Kaptan, K., Beyan, C., Ural, A. U., Cetin, T., Avcu, F., Gulsen, M., Finci, R., & Yalcin, A. (2000). Helicobacter pylori: Is it a novel causative agent in vitamin B_{12} deficiency. *Archives of Internal Medicine, 160*(9), 1349–1353.

Kastin, D. A., & Buchman, A. L. (2002). Nutrition and gastrointestinal disease. *Current Opinion in Gastroenterology, 18*(2), 221–228.

Mahan, K. L., & Escott-Stump, S. E. (Eds.). (2000). *Krause's food nutrition and diet therapy* (10th ed.) (pp. 92–97). Philadelphia: Saunders.

Malinow, M. R., Bostom, A. G., & Krauss, R. M. (1999). Homocysteine, diet, and cardiovascular disease: A statement for healthcare professionals from the nutrition committee, American Heart Association. *Circulation, 99*(1), 178–182.

McCool, A. C., Huls, A., Peppones, M., & Schlenker, E. (2001). Nutrition for older persons: A key to healthy aging. *Topics in Clinical Nutrition, 17*(1), 52–71.

McNally, P. R. (2001). *GI/liver secrets* (2nd ed.) (pp. 332–333). Philadelphia: Hanley & Belfus Publishers.

Shils, M. E., Olson, J. A., Shike, M., & Ross, A. C. (Eds.). (1999). *Modern nutrition in health and disease* (9th ed.) (pp. 869–879). Philadelphia: Lippincott.

Smith, D. L. (2000). Anemia in the elderly. *American Family Physician, 62*(7), 1565–1574.

Snow, C. F. (1999). Laboratory diagnosis of vitamin B_{12} and folate deficiency: A guide for the primary care physician. *Archives of Internal Medicine, 159*(12), 1289–1298.

Tierney, L. M., McPhee, S. J., & Papadakis, M. A. (2000). *Current medical diagnosis & treatment* (39th ed.) (pp. 505–507). New York: McGraw-Hill.

Ulrich, S. P., & Canale, S. W. (2001). *Nursing care planning guidelines* (pp. 79–82). Philadelphia: Saunders.

Verhaar, M. C., Stroes, E., & Rabelink, T. J. (2002). Folates and cardiovascular disease. *Arteriosclerosis, Thrombosis, and Vascular Biology, 22*(1), 6–13.

Cancers of the Gastrointestinal Tract

Ann Schmidt Luggen

The predominant cancers of the GI tract are oropharyngeal, esophageal, stomach, gallbladder, pancreas, liver, small intestine, colon, and rectal. Colorectal cancers have received the most attention because they are so common in elderly people. Emphasis has been placed on screening and new modalities for diagnosis and staging have been developed. There are new treatment regimens (Sial & Catalano, 2001) and palliative techniques. However, we have only begun to understand the complexity of causation and the multiple factors involved in cancer development.

GI neoplasms are a devastating group of malignancies because they present most often in the advanced stages of disease (Hidalgo, 2001). In general, these cancers are resistant to chemotherapy and radiation therapy and are associated with poor prognoses and low survival rates. It is important then, as practitioners who care for elderly clients, to carry out screening activities and maintain a high level of awareness in order that we may diagnose these malignancies earlier and provide a better outcome for our patients.

DEFINITIONS

Cancer is not a single disease and it can affect multiple systems. There are many types (about 100) that differ by organ and also by different cells within the organ. They also differ in severity and in treatment requirements (Novartis Foundation, 2002). Differentiating factors include:

- Type of cell affected
- Hormone involvement
- Speed of cancer cell replication
- How invasive and how metastasisable the cell

CANCERS OF THE ORAL CAVITY

Definition. The oral cavity includes the mouth and oropharynx, the lips, the lining inside the lips and cheeks (buccal mucosa), the teeth, the mouth floor, and the area under the tongue. It includes the hard palate which is the bony top of the mouth, the gums, and the small area behind the wisdom teeth. It also includes the tongue, the soft palate, tonsils, and back of the throat (hypopharynx). It also includes the salivary glands. Squamous cells line the oral cavity. Almost all oral cancers (> 90%) are squamous cell carcinomas (Beers & Berkow, 2000).

Epidemiology. Estimates of new oral cavity cancers for 2002 are 28,900 cases for the U.S. and mortality of 7,400 (American Cancer Society (ACS), 2002). Males have twice the number of oral cavity cancers compared with females and most occur in the later years. However, mortality rates have declined since the 1970s. About one-half of cases occur in those over 65. Survival is high for the first year—84%. The 5-year survival rate is 54%, and the 10-year survival rate is 39%.

The natural course of oral cancers is lymphatic spread. Early areas for detection of spread are the lymph nodes in the neck. It can spread farther, and even if it occurs in the inguinal nodes, it is still classified as the original (primary) oral cancer.

Risk factors. The risk factors should be ascertained from the patient's health history. The risk factors implicated in oral cavity cancers are:

- Cigarette, cigar, or pipe smoking
- Smokeless tobacco, chewing tobacco, dipping snuff
- Betel nut chewing (less common in the U.S.)
- Alcohol consumption, especially if combined with smoking
- Tobacco use accounts for 80–90% of oral cancers, especially smokeless tobacco
- Cancer of the lip may be caused by sun exposure, especially in pipe smokers

- A negative risk factor may be diets that are high in fruits and vegetables (Miller, 1996; ACS, 2002; MedicineNet, 2002).

Signs and symptoms. When assessing the patient, the signs and symptoms to actively look for include:

- A sore that bleeds easily and does not heal
- A lump or thickening on or under the skin
- A red or white patch that persists and cannot be easily scraped off
- Difficulty chewing, swallowing, or moving the jaw or tongue are late signs (ACS, 2002)

Nursing care. Leukoplakia is often an early first finding during assessment; this is a white patch in the mouth. It is associated with heavy tobacco and alcohol use. It occurs in irritated areas such as the gums and buccal mucosa in smokeless tobacco users and the lower lip of pipe smokers (MedicineNet, 2002). Erythroplakia, a red patch in the mouth, occurs most often in elders 60–70. These are premalignant and should be diagnosed and treated early.

Major care of the patient will be reserved for the various specialty oncologists. The advanced practice nurse will refer the patient to a gastroenterologist or a specialist in head and neck. The bedside nurse will request that a physician see the patient. The nurse will anticipate that the patient will have radiation therapy and surgery, and chemotherapy if the malignancy is advanced.

Nursing diagnoses and plan of care. Nursing diagnoses that may be anticipated upon return of the patient to the nurse's care:

- Fear related to cancer diagnosis
- Dry mouth due to radiation therapy
- Sore mouth and throat due to surgery, radiation, and chemotherapy
- Sores in the mouth and GI tract as a result of chemotherapy or infection
- Risk of infection due to cancer therapy
- Decreased quality of life due to inability to taste, chew, swallow, etc.
- Decreased quality of life due to pain
- Loss of self esteem due to physical changes from surgery and radiation

Diagnosis. Usually the diagnosis will be squamous cell carcinoma if cancer is present. The physician will then stage the cancer. This includes dental X-rays of the head and chest. A CT scan may be performed. Ultrasonography, high frequency sound waves (humans cannot hear them) bounce off organs and tissue, and the sound patterns produce the sonogram. An MRI (magnetic resonance imaging) is another tool that may be used in diagnosis. Lymph nodes will be carefully examined for swelling or other changes. A complete physical exam is performed (MedicineNet, 2002).

Interventions, treatments, alternative therapies. The treatment of oral cancer depends on the location, size, type, and extent of the tumor, stage of the disease, as well as the age and health of the patient. A biopsy is the only way to know whether an abnormality is cancer, therefore, the patient is referred to an oral surgeon or ENT specialist. The pathologist will examine the tissue microscopically. The team who will be part of treatment includes the oral surgeon, an ENT surgeon, a medical oncologist, a radiation oncologist, a prosthodontist, a dentist, a plastic surgeon, a dietician, a nurse, and a speech therapist. Most or all of these will be involved in the patient's care.

The older adult will need to be prepared for the team approach to care. For some older adults this process could be overwhelming, while for others it might be a reason for rejecting treatment options and beginning plans for end-of-life or comfort care. The importance of discussing all options with older adults is paramount. Reactions by the older adult may range from opting to not tell significant others or family members, to wanting all significant others to be actively involved in managing care. The provider will need to sensitively support the person's choice.

Surgery will often come first to remove the malignancy and surrounding area. If there is evidence of spread, local lymph nodes may also be removed. If there are further metastases to muscles and other neck tissues, more extensive surgery will be required—perhaps a radical neck dissection. The patient's face may become swollen after surgery. This dissipates in a month or two. However, if there is removal of lymph nodes, this lymph fluid may collect in surrounding tissues and last indefinitely (CancerNet, 2002).

Radiation therapy (RT) may be given before or after surgery and will be localized to the affected area. External radiation is usually required, but radioactive materials or seeds (internal radiation) may be placed in the area of the tumor. In the case of internal radiation, the patient will be somewhat isolated and visiting restricted to short visits. The nurse also will be in the patient's room only briefly for several days. Radiation is sometimes used instead of surgery for small mouth tumors (MedicineNet, 2002).

Radiation treatments are usually given 5 days each week for 6 weeks. New protocols for radiation therapy are trying twice daily RT to determine the effect. The clinical trials are also examining hyperthermia (heat) with "radiosensitizer" drugs to make cells more sensitive to RT.

Aftereffects of radiation therapy may include cracked lips, sore mouth, decreased saliva, and changes in the saliva such that chewing and swallowing become difficult. Mouth dryness promotes tooth decay, so good mouth care is essential. A special toothbrush may be recommended by the dentist consultant who may also prescribe artificial saliva. The dryness may resolve or be permanent. Dentures cannot be worn during this time and possibly for up to a year after RT (MedicineNet, 2002). The dentures may no longer fit after this period of time and replacement may be necessary.

Skin problems are common after radiation therapy. The treated area may become permanently darkened, red, dry, tender, itchy and later, moist and weeping. Protection from sun exposure is very important at this time, although exposure to air is helpful to promote healing (MedicineNet, 2002). The radiologist can recommend moisturizing lotion or ointment that can be applied to the sensitive skin surrounding the marked radiation area. As long as the identification markings are not removed, this skin treatment can reduce the tender and itchy skin. Some lotions or ointments will need to be removed just prior to radiation, but can be reapplied afterward.

Chemotherapy. Side effects of chemotherapy depend on the type of drug given. Common side effects include loss of appetite, nausea, vomiting, mouth sores, and lowered resistance to infection. Older adults seem to suffer less nausea and vomiting from chemotherapy compared with younger patients.

Reconstructive surgery. Often after oral cancer therapy, the patient may need reconstructive and plastic surgery to rebuild bone and tissue. If the elder is not a good candidate for this rehabilitative process, a prosthodontist may be able to make a prosthesis. Usually, the patient will need speech therapy; this will probably continue for some time even after the patient returns home.

Eating problems are common during and after treatment for oral cancer. Considerations for the nurse managing this patient includes teaching the patient to:

- Eat meals and snacks with protein and calories
- Appetites are usually better in the morning; eat more then or have the main meal early in the day and liquid meal replacements later when the patient does not feel hungry or interested in foods

- When the patient is not feeling well, determine what few foods he/she will eat and stick with those until feeling better; use a liquid meal replacement for extra calories and protein
- Some days the patient will not eat at all; make sure he/she tells you if this continues for more than 2–3 days
- Drink plenty of fluids especially on the days when eating seems impossible; try for 6–8 glasses of water or liquid each day; suggest carrying a water bottle around wherever they go (CancerNet, 2002)

Dry Mouth is a problem after radiation and chemotherapy to the head and neck. Foods become harder to chew and swallow. There may be changes in the taste of foods. Considerations for the nurse managing the elder include:

- Carry a water bottle and sip every few minutes to assist in swallowing and in talking; even those wheelchair bound can carry a bottle attached to the vehicle or in a carryall bag attached to the chair.
- Eat very sweet or tart foods and drinks, for example, lemonade; these foods will make use of the salivary gland function that exists; this is not advised if the mouth is sore.
- Suck on hard candy or popsicles, or chew gum; these also produce more saliva.
- Eat soft and pureed foods or mashed potato-like foods which are easier to swallow.
- Moisten foods with sauces, gravies, and salad dressings
- Use lip salves to keep the lips moist
- There are "artificial salivas" that the dentist or specialist may prescribe (CancerNet, 2002)

Sore mouth and tender gums as well as sore throat and esophagus are common problems after surgery and radiation therapies. Certain foods will aggravate this problem and some will make eating easier. Considerations for the nurse managing the patient with this problem include:

- Soft foods such as milkshakes, applesauce, bananas, cottage cheese, yogurt, mashed potatoes, pudding, scrambled eggs or other cooked eggs, and oatmeal.
- Avoid the following foods that will aggravate the pain: citrus fruits, tomato sauces, salty foods, raw vegetables, granolas, and mouthwashes with alcohol

- Cook all foods until soft and tender
- Cut foods into very small pieces
- Use the blender or food processor to make small pieces or to puree
- Mix foods with sauces, gravy, or butter to make it easier to swallow
- Drink liquids with a straw
- Hot foods are irritating; eat cool foods or at room temperature
- Warm bouillon is soothing to a sore throat
- Suck ice chips or popsicles
- Consult with the dentist; he may have a special product for cleaning teeth
- Rinse mouth frequently to remove food and prevent bacterial growth
- Try anesthetic lozenges or sprays to use just while eating meals. (CancerNet, 2002)

Alternative therapies. Mistletoe, a parasitic plant, known best at the winter holiday season, has been shown to kill cancer cells in the laboratory and stimulate the immune system (National Cancer Institute (NCI), 2002). However, in animal studies, there have been mixed results in studies investigating mistletoe's ability to slow tumor growth. Further, both the plant and its berries are toxic to humans.

Coenzyme Q10 is another alternative therapy thought to benefit those with cancer. It is used by cells to produce energy for cell growth and maintenance; it is an antioxidant (NCI, National Center for Complementary and Alternative Medicine, 2002). It is found in most body tissues but mainly in the heart, liver, kidneys, and pancreas. It was discovered in 1958 and researchers found that it was deficient in patients with cancer. It has been tested in humans. The studies have been small but it appears that the drug can cause tumor regression and even remission in some cancers, including GI cancers. The drug is produced and distributed as a nutritional supplement.

Shiitake mushrooms are used as an adjuvant therapy during chemotherapy for some GI cancers. The mushrooms contain a powerful antitumor polysaccharide called lentinan (Boock, 2000). It is effective in helping suppress cancer recurrence. It also seems to lower blood cholesterol and reduce the incidence of blood clots.

Health promotion and quality of life issues. The American Cancer Society has published the following 2015 Goals and Objectives:

- 50% decrease in cancer mortality
- 25% decrease in cancer incidence

- Measurable improvement in quality of life
- Decrease to 12% the number of adults using tobacco products
- Increase to 75% the number of adults consuming more fruits and vegetables
- Increase to 60% the number of adults who increase their levels of physical activity
- Increase to 75% the proportion who use protective measures to decrease skin cancers (ACS, 2002-b.)

There is a major initiative underway to help Americans stop smoking. Initiatives the nurse may take include counseling for smoking cessation in the periodic health examination. While there is no promotional guideline for alcohol cessation, the nurse should ask about alcohol consumption and explain the consequences of continuing to imbibe a moderate to excessive amount. These are major risk factors for oral, laryngeal, and esophageal cancers.

Follow-up care. Nearly 41% of current smokers have tried to quit at least one day in the previous year (ACS, 2002-b). Nearly 23% of U.S. adults are former smokers. It can be done. It may be something that has to be continually addressed in patient care settings.

We usually talk to patients with cancer in terms of remission, rather than cure. Many patients with oral cancer have recovered completely. However, cancer can recur and patients should be assessed on a regular basis for recurrence.

People who have had oral cancer are at increased risk for further oral cancers in another part of the mouth or head or neck. Some research has shown that a substance related to Vitamin A may prevent new cancers (MedicineNet, 2002).

Dental examinations should occur three times each year after oral surgery. The dentist will look for return of the cancer and work to prevent tooth decay, a consequence of the cancer therapy.

There are often dietary problems after oral cancer therapy. Some foods cause pain and patients are likely to lose weight. The rate of survival is low after cancer therapy when there is weight loss. Further, the quality of life is diminished with continuing weight loss and malnutrition. Not only has the elder lost the pleasure of eating, but there is considerable fatigue with malnutrition (Wilkes, 2000).

The patient will need follow-up to observe for depression. After any cancer diagnosis, there is fear of tests, of treatments, of hospitalization, of pain, and of dying. Continuing activities of daily living may be difficult.

If there are changes in appearance, social activities may also diminish. The nurse who is sensitive to these possibilities will look for depression, often missed in older people.

Programs. There are a number of programs available to assist patients with cancer. The ACS can help you and your patients to find them in the region. Two well-known programs are:

- Look Good . . . Feel Better—this is a free program designed to teach women cancer patients beauty techniques to help restore their appearance and self-image.
- I Can Cope—the patient and family receive educational opportunities from a series of classes, usually at local hospitals. Leadership in this program includes physicians, nurses, social workers, and community representatives who provide information about cancer therapy and coping with the challenges of the cancer diagnosis.

Information about oral cancer specifically is available from several sources, such as:

- Cancer Information Service (CIS) 1-800-4-CANCER—this is a program of the National Cancer Institute for patients, families, friends, the public, and health care professionals. Responses are in English and Spanish. Booklets are available.
- American Cancer Society (ACS) 1-800-ACS-2345—this is a voluntary organization with a national office and local units over the entire country. It supports research, conducts educational programs, and offers many services to patients, families, and health care providers.
- National Institutes of Dental Research (see Internet)—this is an agency of the federal government concerned with causes, prevention, diagnosis, and treatment of oral diseases. It has resources such as free booklets and information about oral health after cancer therapy.

CANCERS OF THE ESOPHAGUS

Definition. The esophagus is a tube connecting the throat with the stomach. It lies between the trachea or windpipe, and the spine. It is about 10 inches long. It contains muscles in the walls to push food to the stomach. It contains glands which produce mucus, keeping the passage moist and making swallowing easy. The esophagus is made up of many types of cells. Cancer may develop in any of these different types.

Epidemiology. This disease is common in many areas of the world, but relatively uncommon in the U.S. where it accounts for about 4% of cancers (Beers & Berkow, 2000). About 12,300 Americans were diagnosed with this cancer in 2000, with 12,100 deaths (Mayer, 2002) and it is increasing dramatically. It is common in China, central Asia, South Africa and Latin America. There are isolated pockets of cases in Finland, Iceland, northern France, and Curacao. Fewer than 10% of esophageal tumors are benign. When it spreads outside the esophagus, it appears in nearby lymph nodes, the trachea, the major blood vessels of the chest, and other nearby organs. Late metastases include the lungs, liver, and stomach (MedicineNet-b, 2002). Cancer of the esophagus usually cannot be cured unless found early. Early cancers cause few to no symptoms.

Risk factors. Smoking and excessive use of alcohol are the major risk factors for esophageal cancers. Less known is the risk factor of long-term irritation of esophageal tissues. Patients who have gastroesophageal reflux disease (GERD) are also at risk. Chronic reflux leading to Barrett's esophagus is a risk factor for adenocarcinoma (Mayer, 2002). Other irritants causing cancer are chronic thermal injury such as drinking hot tea, coffee, and soups, and ingestion of caustic substances such as lye. Nitrates (converted to nitrites) are implicated as are fungal toxins in vegetables (Mayer, 2002). Poor nutrition is another factor that increases risk. While it is not known how this risk factor increases the incidence, it is recommended that patients eat fruits and vegetables. Often patients who develop esophageal cancer have no clear risk factors.

Esophageal cancer occurs more commonly in blacks, about 3 times more than in non-Hispanic Whites (NIH, 2002). It occurs predominantly in men (3–5 times more than in women), and smokers. Mortality increases with age, with 66 as the median age at death (Beers & Berkow, 2000).

Signs and symptoms. Small tumors of the esophagus cause no symptoms. As it grows, the patient notes a disturbance in swallowing. They may describe a feeling of fullness, pressure, or burning, as food goes down the esophagus (MedicineNet-b, 2002). The food seems to be "stuck" with increased pressure behind the sternum. Foods most commonly causing symptoms are meat, bread, and raw vegetables. As the esophagus continues to narrow, even liquids become difficult to swallow. Other symptoms reported from patients with esophageal cancer are indigestion, heartburn, frequent choking on foods, hoarseness, and vomiting. Weight loss is common.

Nursing care. The astute nurse will suspect the diagnosis from the description of symptoms and from follow-up on weight loss. Because symptoms occur late in the course of the cancer, the nurse must look for the cause of the symptoms and refer the patient to the specialist. The patient will be referred to a gastroenterologist. The nurse will be involved in following the patient and assessing the weight, swallowing problems, fear, and depression, and in managing the many side effects of therapy.

Nursing diagnoses and plan of care. Nursing diagnoses that may be anticipated with the elderly patient with esophageal cancer include:

- Weight loss due to the inability to swallow
- Fear due to the cancer diagnosis
- Depression due to the change in activities of daily living
- Weakness due to cancer therapy

See Oral Cancer for nursing management as it is very similar to esophageal cancer management.

Diagnosis. In addition to a complete physical examination, chest X-rays and laboratory tests will be ordered. A barium swallow esophagram is a series of X-rays that will show where the swallowing difficulties are by the change in shape of the esophagus. Fluoroscopy is used to watch the barium move down the esophagus to the stomach. Most patients should anticipate having an endoscopy or esophagoscopy. A thin, flexible, lighted instrument is passed through the mouth, down the throat into the esophagus. Biopsies can be taken in the suspicious area for pathology review.

Cancers that occur in the upper and middle part of the esophagus are usually squamous cell carcinoma. These are caused by smoking and alcohol intake. Cancer in the lower esophagus is usually adenocarcinoma (MedicineNet-b, 2002). Staging is done to assist in treatment decisions. About 50% of patients have advanced disease at diagnosis (Beers & Berkow, 2000).

Endoscopy with ultrasound is useful for staging. Often a CT scan of the chest and upper abdomen will be ordered. An MRI scan may also be useful in staging. Laryngoscopy may be performed to see if the cancer has spread to the larynx. Bronchoscopy may be performed to examine the trachea and bronchi. If lymph nodes are enlarged, they will probably be biopsied to look for metastases.

Interventions, treatments, alternative therapies. As in other GI cancers, the patient is usually treated with surgery, radiation therapy, and/or chemotherapy, depending on whether the patient is a good candidate for these therapeutic options. A patient who is frail, or has malnutrition, and other concomitant diseases may not be a candidate for surgery or chemotherapy. The overall cure rate is about 5% although in the distal esophagus, some report a 25% survival rate (Beers & Berkow, 2000).

Surgery is the best treatment for limited tumors and elderly patients do as well as younger patients. However, they suffer a higher incidence of postoperative cardiopulmonary problems (Beers & Berkow, 2000). An esophagectomy is performed, removing the area of involved esophagus and nearby lymph nodes and tissue. The stomach is connected to the remaining esophagus. The surgeon may form a new passage from throat to stomach using tissue from the colon or other part of the digestive tract (MedicineNet-b, 2002).

For those who are not surgical candidates, the surgeon may simply dilate the esophagus. This needs to be repeated as the tumor grows. A tube can be inserted into the esophagus to maintain its dilation. A more recent procedure involves the use of a laser to kill the cancer tissue and relieve blockage.

Radiation therapy (and chemotherapy) may be used prior to surgery, or after surgery, depending on the protocol being used. RT may be used to shrink the tumor prior to surgery especially if the size or location makes surgery more difficult (MedineNet-b, 2002). RT also may be used for palliation of pain and to make swallowing easier. RT alone, in clinical trials, shows poor results in terms of survival. Elders who have RT are at risk for complications. Strictures and fistulas can occur after radiation.

Chemotherapy may be used prior to surgery to reduce tumor mass or after cancer returns when the patient has had surgery and radiation. In general, the goal is to alleviate symptoms, such as malignant dysphagia, and to improve the chances of survival (Fidias, 2001). Drugs commonly used alone and in combination include cisplatin, bleomycin, vindesine, 5-FU, interferon, paclitaxel, irinotecan, epirubicin, and etoposide. The conclusion drawn at the 37th Annual Meeting of the American Society of Clinical Oncology (Hidalgo, 2001) was that patients with resectable esophageal carcinoma benefit from two courses of preoperative chemotherapy and the standard of care should be ECF (epirubicin, cisplatin and 5-FU).

Newer treatment modalities include drug sensitizers for radiation therapy. Photodynamic therapy using laser light combined with drugs that make cells sensitive to laser therapy is recent. Laser therapy followed by brachytherapy (intraluminal placement of radioactive materials into the esophagus via a nasogastric applicator) is an option for palliation of advanced esophageal cancers and for those who are not candidates for other therapies. Most patients in one trial were able to eat a soft diet and sometimes solids after the treatment (Spencer, 2002). Biologicals to increase the immune system are in clinical trials.

Dietary deficiencies of zinc, vitamin A, and molybedenum have been implicated in the causation of esophageal cancer, although there is no strong data to support it fully. It is likely that therapy with vitamin A and other supplements will be tried by many.

Health promotion and quality of life issues. See Oral Cancers. Like oral cancers, esophageal cancers are devastating to the patient, and to the family and others involved in care. Self-help groups and meeting with other similar patients can be helpful in coping with this disease and the effects of therapy.

Risk factors for esophageal cancer have been identified, although the exact cause is not known. Stopping smoking and drinking alcohol must be strongly encouraged.

Much can be done to help the patient eat, both from a nursing and a medical viewpoint. This should be actively done so that the patient does not become malnourished and fatigued and less able to deal with infections and other side effects of cachexia.

GASTRIC CANCERS

The stomach is part of the digestive system located in the abdomen under the ribs. Stomach (gastric) cancer can develop in any part of the stomach and may spread throughout the stomach and to other organs (Cancer.gov, 2002). It may grow along the stomach wall into the esophagus or small intestine.

Epidemiology. Gastric cancers were the most common forms of cancer in the world in the 1970s and 1980s (Cancer.gov, 2002). It is now surpassed only by lung cancer. There is substantial variation internationally—highest in Japan, eastern Asia, eastern Europe, and parts of Latin America.

In the U.S. there were 22,000 new cases and 14,000 deaths each year, in 1999 (Beers & Berkow, 2000). Over 70% of these affect adults over the age of 65.

It is believed that the recent decline of gastric cancers in the world is due to better techniques in food preservation and storage. There is evidence that high salt intake is a major determinant of risk. Since refrigeration has become more prevalent, fewer foods are salted and smoked and more fresh fruits and vegetables are eaten.

Benign tumors of the stomach are common, especially in older adults (Beers & Berkow, 2000). These are hyperplastic and adenomatous polyps. Hyperplastic polyps are nonmalignant, however, adenomatous polyps greater than 2 cm have malignant potential.

Risk factors. Ethnic groups at highest risk for gastric cancer are Koreans, Vietnamese, Japanese, Alaska Natives, and Hawaiians. At intermediate risk are White, Hispanic, Chinese, and Black populations (Cancer.gov, 2002). Risk is similar in men and women.

The most important risk factor for gastric cancer is Helicobacter pylori (Beers & Berkow, 2000). H. pylori is also associated with a low-grade gastric lymphoma. Having gastric ulcers alone does not increase the risk unless accompanied by H. pylori. Other risk factors include adenomas, chronic atrophic gastritis with intestinal metaplasia (with or without pernicious anemia), adenomatous polyps, and chronic gastric ulcers. The relative risk of acquiring gastric adenocarcinoma with pernicious anemia is 3 times higher than that of age-matched controls (Beers & Berkow, 2000). Other suspected risk factors are dusts and fumes in the workplace and smoking (Medicine-net-c, 2002).

Signs and symptoms. Usually, gastric cancers are without early symptoms. Vague epigastric discomfort is common as the presenting symptom, followed by anorexia and early satiety (Beers & Berkow, 2000). Later signs and symptoms are nausea, vomiting, dysphagia, hematemesis, melena, severe abdominal pain, weight loss, palpable mass, and lymph node enlargement.

Nursing care. It is important that nurses be aware that a positive H. pylori test increases the risk of a gastric cancer. In one study, both strongly positive and weakly positive (fewer in the negative) groups had a high risk for gastric cancer (Yamaji, 2002). In subjects age 60 or older, the weakly positive H. pylori antibody test showed the highest risk. Vague symptoms are the only symptoms, if any, early in gastric cancer. A high index of suspicion is warranted with persistent vague symptoms.

After gastrectomy, patients are unable to absorb vitamin B12 and will need regular injections of this vitamin (Cancer.gov, 2002). They may be unable to eat their usual foods and have to change their diet. Patients will begin with liquids, then soft foods, then solids. Some patients will not be able to advance to solids and diet change will be permanent.

Patients may have dumping syndrome, which consists of cramping, nausea, diarrhea, and dizziness after eating because the food enters the small intestine too quickly. Food high in sugar are especially problematic. Nurses advise patients to eat small, frequent meals throughout the day. Encourage protein intake for healing. Fluids will be discouraged during the mealtimes as this would also hasten the dumping. This problem may slowly dissipate, but it can be permanent.

See the Oral Cancers section of this chapter for management of radiation therapy problems and side effects. All the therapies including biologicals have side effects that will require management. Most patients will be fatigued and nauseated, and with biologicals may have chills and fever. When severe, the patient needs to remain in the hospital.

Nursing diagnoses and plan of care. These will be similar to the previous cancers described earlier in the chapter.

Diagnosis. The patient will have a complete physical examination, review of the medical history, and laboratory studies, such as:

- Fecal occult blood test (FOBT) for hidden blood in the stool
- Upper GI Series (UGI) of the esophagus and stomach using a barium swallow.
- Endoscopy, performed by a gastroenterologist for direct observation of the stomach, and possible biopsy.

Adenocarcinoma accounts for 95% of all stomach cancers (Beers & Berkow, 2000). It is found more in Blacks and men (2:1), compared with women.

Interventions, treatments, alternative therapies. If cancer is found by the pathologist, staging the disease will follow. Stomach cancer often spreads to the liver, pancreas, and lungs, and the cancer specialist will order a CT scan, an ultrasound exam, and other tests to determine the extent of spread. Staging won't be complete until after surgery (MedicineNet-c, 2002) in which lymph nodes are taken and samples of tissue in other areas of the abdomen. The results will determine treatment and management.

The overall 5-year survival rate for gastric adenocarcinoma is less than 10%. If early gastric cancer is found, 5-year survival rates are reported up to 95% (Beers & Berkow, 2000).

Surgery. Gastrectomy is the most common treatment for gastric cancer (Cancer.gov, 2002). This may be total or subtotal (partial). The surgeon will connect the remaining stomach to the esophagus or small intestine. With a total gastrectomy, the esophagus will be connected directly to the small intestine. Lymph nodes nearby will be removed to assess for cancer cells.

Radiation therapy. RT may be given prior to surgery to shrink the tumor, after surgery in combination with chemical therapy, or during surgery as intraoperative radiation therapy.

Chemotherapy. As with other GI cancers, this may be given prior to surgery to shrink the tumor or after surgery. Advanced cancer may be treated with 5-FU, methotrexate, and adriamycin or mitomycin. Another regimen includes cisplatin and CPT-11 or 5-FU/leucovorin and Cpt-11 (Hidalgo, 2001). Combination therapy with RT is often used. Intraperitoneal chemotherapy, in which chemicals are placed directly into the abdomen, is being studied in clinical trials.

Biologicals. Immunotherapy is a form of treatment that helps the immune system destroy cancer cells. At this time, biologicals are being used in clinical trials to prevent recurrence of gastric cancers. Colony-stimulating factors are another form of biological therapy used to restore low blood counts that occur frequently during or after chemotherapy (Cancer.gov, 2002).

Health promotion and quality of life issues. Because this cancer, like other GI cancers, is detected so late in the disease course, planning for end-of-life issues should be discussed early with the elderly patient and family, when appropriate (Beers & Berkow, 2000).

Palliative surgery for late stage gastric cancer produces high complication rates. Therefore, palliative surgical procedures should only be performed in those with few comorbid conditions, and with good function. Palliation with endoscopic laser photoablation may be useful in those with esophageal or gastric outlet obstruction (Beers & Berkow, 2000).

End-of-life symptoms with gastric cancer are very difficult for patients and family. Nausea, vomiting, pain, and weight loss are all common and a strong effort of all the health care team needs to be made to control symptoms.

Follow-up care. Close follow-up for metastases is warranted since most gastric cancers are found late in the course. In addition to extension and lymph node involvement, the liver, pancreas, esophagus, and colon are common sites. Distant sites include the lungs, supraclavicular lymph nodes, and ovaries (Medicine-net-c, 2002). Patients who have had chemotherapy will be subject to infections and the family and elder must be taught to look for these. There may be hair loss and poor self image, and depression may develop. Preparation for these occurrences should be in place.

Nutrition is an important issue in follow-up with elderly patients. There will be loss of appetite and often nausea. They feel full after eating only a very small amount of food. Taste changes that occur with aging emphasize the problem.

See the followup of previous cancers in this chapter for additional care. Resources include the National Cancer Institute booklet, *Eating Hints for Cancer Patients* and *Taking Time* (for the family) from the Cancer Information Service. Call 1-800-4-CANCER for these and other helpful booklets.

COLORECTAL AND ANAL CANCERS

The colon and rectum are part of the digestive system forming a long muscular tube; the first 4-1/2 to 6 feet of the large intestine is the colon;

the last 8–10 inches is the rectum. The anus is the last segment and meets the exterior skin at its margin. Cancer affecting these organs is colorectal cancer. Cancer of the anus is often discussed separately, since it has different causes.

Definition. Colorectal cancer is one of the most preventable cancers and yet is found usually quite late in its course. Most start as polyps on the innermost layer of tissue and produce no symptoms. Therefore, screening is very important especially in adults over 50 years of age.

Epidemiology. Colorectal cancer is second only to lung cancer in causing cancer-related deaths in the U.S. and one in 20 people will develop the disease in their lifetime. New cases in 2002 numbered 148,000 (Jemel, Thomas, Murray, & Thun, 2002). Estimated deaths for 2002 were 56,600. Rectal cancers make up about one-third of the colorectal cancers. Current anal cancer incidence is 3900 new cases and 500 deaths annually. The survival rate for colorectal cancer is 90% if diagnosed early (ACS-c, 2002). Most colorectal cancers (90%) occur in adults over 50 years of age (Russell & Mason, 2000). The incidence increases with age, until age 95 (Balducci, 2002). There is wide divergence by racial and ethnic groups. Rates in the Alaskan native population are four times greater than the American Indian population (NCI, 2002). After Alaskan natives, the next highest rates are in Japanese, Blacks and non-Hispanic Whites, Chinese, Hawaiians, and Vietnamese, followed by White Hispanics, Koreans, and Filipinos. The incidence is low in American Indians in New Mexico (NCI, 2002).

Risk factors. Age is a risk factor as 90% of people diagnosed are over 50. Other factors include:

- Chronic disease of the colon, such as ulcerative colitis (Crohn's disease)
- Race—African Americans have a higher risk than other races
- Family history of colorectal cancer (parent, sibling, child) or adenomatous polyps of the colon
- Familial Polyposis Syndrome
- Personal history of adenomatous colon polyps
- Diets high in fats and low in fiber
- Smoking
- Excessive alcohol intake
- Sedentary lifestyle, perhaps by modulation of hormones

Signs and symptoms. The signs and symptoms of colon cancer for adults and older adults have been well publicized and, fortunately, many Americans are aware and seek medical attention when they occur. This fact and/or the recent emphasis on screening may be responsible for the decreasing incidence of colorectal cancer deaths in recent years. Some of the signs and symptoms are:

- Rectal bleeding or pain
- Change in regular bowel habits
- Unexplained anemia
- Unexplained weight loss
- New onset of lower abdominal pain

Nursing care. It is helpful if the nurse understands the treatment of colorectal cancer and can assist the elder and family in making a decision about therapy. Chemotherapy can be very toxic and one regimen has a 5% death rate (Macdonald, 2001), so patients should understand the possible or probable consequences of therapy. Further, there are different methods of giving chemotherapy—continuous vs. "drug holidays"—the continuous therapy causing more adverse effects and worse quality of life and a shorter survival. It is more helpful in making a decision if as many facts as are known, can be given to those making the decisions.

The nurse may be involved in the preparation for colonoscopy. The patient needs a liquid diet for 1–3 days prior and then a laxative just before the procedure. In the procedure, the patient lies on the left side on the examination table and is given a sedative and pain medication to maintain comfort during the exam. A long, flexible lighted tube is inserted into the rectum and air is blown in to inflate the colon and maintain visibility. Any polyp or inflamed tissue can be removed with tiny instruments through the scope and sent to pathology for biopsy (NIH, 1998). The procedure takes between 30–60 minutes and the patient will be in recovery for 1–2 hours until sedation wears off.

The nurse may need to discuss ostomies with the patient prior to surgery and instruct the elder and family after surgery. Sometimes these are temporary and sometimes permanent; some have one opening and some have two. A good source for information about ostomies is the United Ostomy Association at *www.uoa.org/ostomyinfo.shtml*

Elders receiving chemotherapy will experience many common side effects such as diarrhea, mucositis (sore mouth), and low blood counts, especially in older adults (Savarese, 2001). Nurses should observe for dehydration with diarrhea. Palmar-plantar-dysesthesias (soreness, redness, and peeling skin on the palms and soles of the feet) occurs with oral 5-FU.

Some of the surgeries for colorectal/anal cancers may involve the anal sphincter. These surgeries and management of recurrences in the area cause profound morbidity and suffering (Ryan, 2001).

One of the problems patients have following colectomy is postoperative recovery of gastrointestinal function and resumption of oral intake. Opioids are necessary to maintain patient comfort but contribute to the delay in recovery. A new investigational drug, ADL8-2698, in a study published in New England Journal of Medicine (Taguchi et al., 2001) seems to allow significantly faster recovery while allowing for opioids for postoperative pain relief. The median time to passage of flatus decreased from 70 to 49 hours; time to first bowel movement decreased from 111 hours to 70 hours and patients were able to be discharged earlier.

Nursing diagnoses and plan of care. See this section in Oral Cancers.

Diagnoses. The diagnosis is obtained after a full clinical workup (Balducci, 2002). This usually consists of colonoscopy, CT scan of the abdomen and pelvis, and a PET (positron emission tomography) scan if available. The addition of PET scanning can affect the basic management and is a useful tool for diagnosis and staging (Macdonald, 2001). A CEA (carcinoembryonic antigen) lab test is obtained prior to surgery for data when looking for recurrences. Diagnosis is made from the biopsy specimen taken at the time of colonoscopy.

Staging is done to plan for appropriate therapy. The following are the stages of cancer of the colon (Balducci, 2002) and the 5-year survival rate, based on stage at diagnosis (Healthandage, 2002):

- I: Disease limited to mucosa and submucosa—90%+
- IIA: Involvement of muscularis propria—85%
- IIB: Involvement of the serosa—85%
- III: Involvement of regional lymph nodes—70–80%
- IV: Distant metastases—5%
- Recurrence of disease, after treatment

Interventions, treatments, and alternative therapies. Age should not be the major consideration when addressing treatment of colon cancers (Sial & Catalano, 2001). A thorough medical evaluation is necessary to determine risks and optimize outcomes. Some of the common management strategies are presented here. However, there are clinical trials available for elders who wish to pursue this course.

Surgery. Treatment of Stage I and IIA colon cancer with surgical resection will result in a cure rate of about 90% (Balducci, 2002). Some surgeons are opting for laparoscopic surgery, which entails a shorter hospital stay and less postoperative pain compared with the standard, open colectomy (Weeks & Nelson, 2002). However, some patients having this procedure also had to have a colectomy. This procedure is still investigational. Rectal cancer with a diameter of ≤ 2.5 cm and less than 1/3 of the rectal wall and depth does not reach the serosa (using ultrasound) will be resected transanally with RT to follow. Rectal cancer is surgically resected and varies based on the extent of disease and location of the tumor. It ranges from transanal excision to pelvic exenteration and includes RT and chemotherapy (Savarese, 2001).

Chemotherapy. For some Stage IIB and III cancers, a combination of 5-FU and leucovorin may be administered over a 6-month period (Balducci, 2002). Metastatic colon cancer may warrant 5-FU, leucovorin, and irinotecan which has a response rate of 40% but a median duration of 8 months. An international team of researchers has analyzed 7 clinical trials and found that adults over 70 do as well with chemotherapy for colon cancer as younger patients (Sargent, 2001). However, these patients were in good physical condition, without multiple chronic illnesses. This data is difficult to apply to patients over 80 years old. Thalidomide is being used in clinical trials at this time for recurrent colorectal cancer and there is no age limit for enrolling (NCI, 2001). The most recent clinical trial for treatment of advanced colorectal cancer is N9741 or the FOLFOX4 regimen. Patients live four months longer than with other therapies, a median of 18.6 months. Patients and physicians can call the NIH about eligibility for this trial at 1-800-4-Cancer.

Biologics. Clinical trials are presently testing anti-EGFR (epidermal growth factor receptor), cetuximab, plus irinotecan results in objective tumor regression in 22.5% of patients refractory to irinotecan chemotherapy. The median duration of response was 186 days (Macdonald, 2001). Immunotherapy, using monoclonal antibody 17-1A is a subject of discussion at the research table.

Other. A team from Japan has investigated the effects of cimetedine in patients with curative surgery. The 10-year survival of the cimetedine group was 85%, and 50% of the control group. Cimetedine seems to inhibit the adhesion of cancer cells to endothelium (Matsumoto, 2002). Further trials of this therapy are needed.

Alternative therapies. Coenzyme Q10 is said to be a therapy for colon cancer because the enzyme was found to be low in cancer patients. It works as an antioxidant and may stimulate the immune system. There are no randomized clinical trials supporting its efficacy (NCI, 2002). Some of the natural medicines that are *possibly effective* include barley, calcium, folic acid, garlic, lutein, melatonin, oats, olive oil, pyridoxine, selenium, vitamin C, and vitamin E (Jellin, 2002).

Palliative therapies. There are a number of palliative treatments available for late-stage colon cancer with liver metastases. Cryoablation, ultrasound, radiofrequency ablation, regional infusional therapy, and chemotherapeutic agents delivered locally with surgically implanted pumps are some that are used (Fong, 1999), although some of these may still be investigational.

Health promotion and quality of life issues. Prevention of colorectal cancer is of considerable interest to researchers and this form of cancer is considered highly preventable. It seems to be closely related to dietary intake. The recommended diet is high in fruits, vegetables, and fiber, and low in calories and animal fat (Russell & Mason, 2000). Diet components that appear, but are not proven, to be protective include calcium, vitamin D, aspirin, possibly raisins (high in salicylate), some NSAIDs including the COX-2 inhibitors, folate, vitamin E, fiber, and in particular, the antioxidant selenium. Garlic has not panned out as chemoprotective. Physical activity may be helpful because it prevents obesity with its high circulating insulin levels, or because of its role in modulating hormones. There is some evidence that oral contraceptives and postmenopausal estrogen replacement therapy may be protective against colorectal cancer (Fernandez, 2001). Duration of use does not appear to affect risk.

If there is family history of colon polyps or colon cancer, the older adult at risk should be evaluated with colonoscopy beginning at age 40, or at least 10 years prior to the age that the family member was identified with polyps or cancer.

Screening. Recommendations for screening include annual digital exam starting at age 40, annual fecal occult blood test starting at age 50, and visualization of the colon via colonoscopy (preferred), sigmoidoscopy, or barium enema. It is known that the test for fecal blood is a useful tool for screening for colon cancer. However, information from the American Cancer Society states that only 11.6% of those 50+ from Alabama and 35.8% of those from D.C. have been tested. More women than men have the test performed (ACS, 2002). Sigmoidoscopy or colonoscopy percentages are 22.6% in Nebraska to 42.6% in Delaware. For racial and ethnic groups, screening is highest in White/non-Hispanics, and lowest in American-Indians/Alaska natives (Jemal et al., 2002).

A report from the Agency for Healthcare Research and Quality (AHRQ) (2001) states that screening for colorectal cancer every 5 years reduces mortality at a cost similar to other cancer screening procedures. The most effective strategy is FOBT (fecal occult blood testing) plus sigmoidoscopy, followed by colonoscopy if a polyp is found. This strategy results in a 60% reduction in mortality compared with no screening.

There is also a new screening tool on the horizon. The American Cancer Society (2002-d) described a study looking at a DNA test that can locate a gene called APC which is transformed when colon cancer develops. The screening is performed via colonoscopy and is said to be safe and reliable. Marketing is anticipated by 2004.

Follow-up care. The patient will need sequential measurements of the CEA to allow detection of recurrences of the colon cancer. If the therapy is thought to be curative, there will be follow-up with surveillance colonoscopy (Balducci, 2002). This will occur one year postop, and then at 3–5 year intervals. The consensus of an expert panel is that the patient should have a pertinent physical examination and clinical history every 3–6 months for the first 3 years, then annually (National Institutes of Health, 1998). Fecal occult blood testing, liver function tests, and complete blood counts should be done on a regular basis, also.

Palliative care may be the follow-up care for many elders with colorectal cancer. In one study reported in *Colorectal Disease* (Harris, 2002) of 377 patients (median age 64, 232 males), the operative mortality was 6%, crude 6-month survival was 71%, and median survival was 10.5 months. Significant factors included age. Palliative resection may be warranted with an acceptable mortality rate.

One patient resource is a document entitled *A Patient's Guide: Followup Care for Colorectal Cancer* from the American Society for Clinical Oncology (ASCO) at *guideline@asco.org*

HEPATOCELLULAR AND BILIARY CARCINOMAS

Deaths from hepatocellular and biliary tract carcinomas (gallbladder cancer and cholangiocarcinoma) have increased over the past 3 decades in the U.S. (Nair, 2002). Mortality has doubled in white males and increased modestly in women. The mean age at death in biliary tract cancers has increased from 67 to 73 years. There has been no increase in mortality from HCC in African Americans, however, the number of deaths in this population from biliary tract cancers has doubled.

Definition. Hepatocellular carcinoma (HCC) is a primary tumor of the liver and usually develops in those with chronic liver disease, especially viral hepatitis. HCC accounts for 90% of liver cancers (Beers & Berkow, 2000). Cholangiocarcinoma arises from the epithelial cells of the intrahepatic and extrahepatic bile ducts and is predominantly adenocarcinoma. This cancer is not common in the U.S., accounting for only about 3% of GI cancers, but is highly lethal when it does occur (Lowe, Kim, Chari, & Afdhal, 2001). Gallbladder cancers are usually found at cholecystectomy (surgery for gallstones) (Lazcano-Ponce et al., 2001).

Epidemiology. HCC is one of the most common cancers worldwide, especially in areas where viral hepatitis is common (Beers & Berkow, 2000). In the U.S. HCC has been increasing over the past 20 years, especially in those 40–60 years of age. Older patients with longstanding liver disease are most likely to develop HCC (Schwartz & Carithers, 2001). It is more common in men. Biliary tract cancers increase with age, the typical patient being 50–70 years of age.

The incidence of HCC and BDC is lowest in non-Hispanic Whites. Blacks and Hispanic populations have an incidence twice as high as Whites (Miller et al., 1996). The highest incidence is in Chinese, and in Vietnamese men, probably due to the high prevalence of viral hepatitis in China and Vietnam. The 5-year survival for bile duct cancer (BDC) is only 5% and many of the tumors are not operable. Most liver cancer occurs in older age groups except when it occurs in high-risk racial or ethnic groups.

Gallbladder cancer is the fourth most common GI cancer in the U.S.and represents 80–95% of biliary tree cancers. Most GB cancers are adenocarcinoma (80%); others are squamous cell carcinoma and adenoacanthoma. About 85% accompany gallstones. The average age at diagnosis is 76 years (Beers & Berkow, 2000). It occurs more in women over the age of 65, but occurs also in workers in rubber and automobile plants. The 5-year survival rate is 5%. There is a marked regional and ethnic variation in gallbladder cancer, the highest rates in Bolivia and Chile (Lazcano-Ponce et al., 2001). In North America, the Indians of New Mexico have the highest rates.

Risk factors. HCC risk factors have been identified. They include:

• Cirrhosis (any cause) especially with viral hepatitis
• Hepatitis B carrier state
• Environmental toxins—molds (aflatoxin) in stored foods and peanuts in Africa and Asia; liver parasites in southeast Asia; industrial vinyl chloride exposure (Miller et al., 1996); contaminated drinking water; betel nut chewing; cigarette smoking (Schwartz & Carithers, 2001)
• Chronic hepatitis C virus (HCV) infection
• Hereditary hemochromatosis (Schwartz & Carithers, 2001)

Predisposing factors for cholangiocarcinoma are:

• Primary sclerosing cholangitis (PSC) and ulcerative colitis
• Choledochal cysts—congenital cysts of the bile ducts
• Parasite infestation with liver flukes causing chronic inflammation

- Industrial exposure—rubber, automobile, chemical, and wood-finishing plants
- Radiologic contrast agent—Thorotrast
- Gallstones (Beers & Berkow, 2000; Lowe, Kim, Chari, & Afdhal, 2001)

Risk factors for gallbladder cancer are:

- Female sex
- Increasing age
- Chronic cholelithiasis (gallstones) with/without GB polyps
- Chronic inflammation and gallbladder infection, especially Salmonella typhi
- Family history of gallstones
- Biliary tract cancer
- High BMI
- Elevated glucose
- Increased parity
- Low HDL cholesterol
- Occupation—workers in oil, paper, chemical, shoe, textile, and cellulose acetate industries, and exposure to radon. (Zakko & Zakko, 2002)

Signs and symptoms. The clinical presentation of HCC usually occurs late in the course of the disease. Abdominal pain from a large tumor is the most common presentation (MedicineNet-d, 2002). Weight loss and fever can be considered warning signs in elders with cirrhosis. Any change in a stable patient with cirrhosis should be a warning. This includes jaundice, ascites, new muscle wasting, encephalopathy, and esophageal varices. A bruit may be heard over the liver with a stethoscope.

Bile duct cancers are symptomatic early in the course of disease; jaundice occurs in nearly all patients (Beers & Berkow, 2000). RUQ pain is common and other signs include nausea, vomiting, weight loss, fever, chills, and liver enlargement. The gallbladder may also be palpable.

The early clinical presentation of gallbladder cancer is an intermittent, vague pain in the RUQ or the epigastrium. Most patients are diagnosed late in the course of the disease and present with weight loss, jaundice, and a tender, firm, palpable mass.

Nursing care. Again, death and dying issues should be appropriately managed in these elderly patients. With a 5-year survival rate of only 5%, clearly end-of-life issues must be addressed. Palliative care may be instituted early since most patients present late in the course of the disease. There is little in the way of therapy for GB cancers. Surgery will be done, but no radiation or chemotherapy, as they are not useful in this disease

In patients receiving intrahepatic chemotherapy, the patient will stay overnight in hospital. The groin is compressed with a sandbag and must be checked regularly for bleeding. The pulse of the foot on the side of the site is also checked to determine patency of the artery (MedicineNet-d, 2002).Patients with gallbladder cancer and cholangiocarcinoma will have a cholecystectomy.

Nursing diagnoses and plan of care. See previous descriptions of GI cancers.

Diagnosis. In HCC liver function tests will be abnormal, probably due to cirrhosis. Serum bilirubin is elevated, as is alkaline phosphatase and y-glutamyl transpeptidase. Serum albumin is diminished (Beers & Berkow, 2000). Diagnosis is confirmed with abdominal ultrasound, MRI, CT scan, angiography, and fine needle biopsy. High-risk patients with cirrhosis may be screened on a regular basis using ultrasound. The tumor marker, AFP (alpha-fetoprotein), is identifiable by a biochemical blood test used widely for screening. However, it is not very sensitive for HCC (60%) (Medi-cineNet-d, 2002). Staging of the cancer will occur. A small solitary tumor has a 90% 1-year survival prognosis even without treatment; 50% for 3 years, 20% for 5 years (MedicineNet-d, 2002).

Ultrasound and CT scan will confirm the diagnosis for bile duct cancers. For tumor localization, percutaneous transhepatic cholangiography and retrograde cholangiopancreatography will be done. The gallbladder (GB) cancer can be visualized with abdominal ultrasound (81%) (Zakko & Zakko, 2002). CT scan is useful for staging GB cancer by revealing liver metastases or invasion. Endoscopic ultrasound has been found to be very useful, although it is not widely available.

Interventions, treatments, alternative therapy.

Surgery. Elders with cirrhosis and liver cancer are not good candidates for surgery. A liver transplant is the only curative therapy, although there are surgeons who will remove the liver tumor without a transplant (Medi-cineNet-d, 2002). With resection, there are likely to be recurrences of HCC. Elders will fare better with transplant than resection.

Some bile duct tumors are not operable. Those that are resectable have greater 5-year survival rates (20–30%) but patients over 70 have a high operative risk (Beers & Berkow, 2000). Most patients with gallbladder cancer are diagnosed at an advanced stage and the 5-year survival rate is

5%; however, if discovered early, at Stage I for example, from pathology reports after cholecystectomy, the 5-year survival rate is 85% (Zakko & Zakko, 2002). In the U.S. cholecystectomy is the most common abdominal surgery; this is probably the reason that the incidence of gallbladder cancer is so low (Lazcano-Ponce et al., 2001).

Radiation therapy. Radiofrequency ablation (RFA) is the therapy of choice in the U.S. (MedicineNet-d, 2002). This causes necrosis of the tumor. There are adverse effects associated with this treatment, however. In one clinical trial, RFA performed better than PEI (see Other, below) and RFA had a better recurrence-free survival at one year and at two years.

Local radiation therapy may be useful in some instances. Those who have failed TACE or have unresectable disease may be candidates (Schwartz, Stuart, & Carithers, 2001).

Chemotherapy. Doxorubicin and 5-FU are commonly used for HCC. Other drugs may be added, such as tamoxifen, octreotide, gemcitabine, and cisplatin. For the most part, results are disappointing (MedicineNet-d, 2002). Intra-arterial infusion into the liver is one method of chemotherapy delivery. However, there are many side effects such as inflammation of the gallbladder or liver failure in those with cirrhosis. TACE, trans-arterial chemoembolization, is a newer technique for chemotherapy infusion. In addition, TACE blocks vessels that "feed" the tumor. There seems to be some success with TACE especially when used prior to transplant; it is also used as a palliative measure.

Biologics. A drug not yet available in the U.S., acyclic retinoids, inhibits hepatocarcinogenesis in the laboratory, and in human tests significantly reduced the incidence of recurrences. Interferon has also been tried. Immunotherapy using recombinant interleukin-2 and anti CD3 antibody has been tried in Japan with some success.

Other. Percutaneous ethanol injections (PEI) into a tumor induces necrosis and tumor shrinkage (Schwartz, Stuart, & Carithers, 2001). This is generally well tolerated but does have some adverse effects. Survival rates are similar to resection.

Alternative therapy. Supplementation with selenium may reduce risk or prevent HCC. Some experimental and epidemiologic studies have linked low selenium levels with HCC (Schwartz, Stuart, & Carithers, 2001).

Health promotion and quality of life issues. Primary prevention strategies are very successful in preventing hepatitis. Immunization against hepatitis B resulted in a 50% decline in incidence of HCC in Taiwan (Schwartz, Stuart, & Carithers, 2001). Immunization is taking place now in 85 countries and should greatly affect the incidence of HCC. Treatment of chronic hepatitis C with interferon is associated with a decline in the risk of developing HCC.

There is no primary prevention for gallbladder cancer since the etiology is unknown (Lazcano-Ponce et al., 2001). However, increasing the availability of laparoscopic cholecystectomy for symptomatic gallstone patients is an effective secondary prevention.

Follow-up and palliative care. See previous description of GI cancers. A program of palliative care assumes that the situation is irreversible and that death will come within a short time (Novartis Foundation for Gerontology, 2002). Goals are to improve the quality of the patient's remaining life and to maintain comfort during the dying process.

In the frail elder, mental well-being may be as important to quality of life as actual health and ability to function. One common reaction is refusing to go to the hospital because that is where people go to die, so by staying at home the patient will avoid death.

Other considerations for palliative care in elderly cancer patients include:

- Treat existing health problems; they may be more troublesome on a daily basis than the cancer
- Find approaches that help the elder deal with denial, disbelief, anger, and resentment before coming to terms with death
- Counsel and help the patient prepare for death in practical ways
- Consider holistic or alternative medicine
- Discuss living wills and how the elder would wish to die
- Provide comfort for relatives who may be in emotional distress
- Suggest support groups for the patient or relatives or caregivers
- Arrange later support for the bereaved
- Involve the patient in decisions about care
- Maintain pain relief
- Assure adequate rest and sleep

PANCREATIC CANCERS

Definition. Pancreatic tumors include exocrine and endocrine types. Endocrine tumors are rare in elders and include insulinomas and gastrinomas, to name two (Beers & Berkow, 2000). More than 75% are exocrine cancers, i.e., adenocarcinomas. Pancreatic cancers are considered the most deadly malignancy and the death/incidence ratio is .99 (Lillemoe, Yeo, & Cameron, 2000).

Epidemiology. According to the American Cancer Society (2002), more than 30,000 new cases of pancreatic cancer were estimated for 2002, contrasted with 7000 new cases of gallbladder and cholangiocarcinomas. Nearly all of these cancers occur in adults older than 65 (Beers & Berkow, 2000), and 80% occur between 60–80 (Lillemoe et al., 2000). Most patients diagnosed with pancreatic cancer will die, with 29,700 deaths expected in 2002. More cases and more deaths occur in women than men. However, the rate is 10 times higher in men at age 75 compared with the general population. Over the past 20 years rates have declined slowly, but pancreatic cancer is the fifth leading cause of cancer death.

Risk factors. Pancreatic cancer rates are highest in countries whose populations eat a high-fat diet. The rate is highest in Western and industrialized countries, and low in underdeveloped nations. Other risk factors include:

- Cigarette and cigar smoking—twice as high as in nonsmokers
- Advancing age
- Jewish religion (in U.S. and in Israel)
- Hereditary—rare
- Black race
- Obesity
- Physical inactivity
- Chronic pancreatitis
- Diabetes—relative risk 2.1 compared with nondiabetics; diabetes may be caused by the pancreatic cancer
- Cirrhosis
- Alcohol and coffee (ACS, 2002; Beers & Berkow, 2000; Lillemoe, Yeo, & Cameron, 2000; Fernandez-del Castillo et al., 2002)

Signs and symptoms. This cancer develops without any early symptoms. If it occurs near the common bile duct, there will be jaundice; in this event, it may be diagnosed early. Later symptoms include dull pain in the upper abdomen that radiates to the back (80–85% of patients) and feels worse when the patient is supine. The pain may be intermittent, and it may be worse with eating (Steer, 2002). Weight loss may be associated with anorexia, early satiety, nausea, steatorrhea, or diarrhea, and may be profound. Other signs may include abdominal mass or ascites (20% of patients). A palpable, nontender gallbladder in the right costal margin may be seen in patients with jaundice. Occasionally the patient will present with a new onset atypical diabetes mellitus (15–20%) or a new or previous attack of pancreatitis. A large nodular liver is a late presentation and indicates metastases.

Nursing care. Patients with jaundice often have pruritis and it is very difficult to find relief. Teach to avoid hot showers and baths, rubbing alcohol, and harsh detergents (Beers & Berkow, 2000). Wash only areas with skin folds and use a mild soap. Antihistamines are useful in some people, but dangerous in elderly people. Different creams and ointments may be tried, but ointments are usually best.

About one-third of patients present with moderate to severe pain. Intractable pain is common with advanced pancreatic cancer (Lillemoe et al., 2000). Pain takes on a life of its own and becomes a problem that is more pressing to the patient than the disease. It causes sleeplessness, depression, isolation, disability, delirium, and profound suffering. The management of intractable pain requires consultation with a pain specialist who has multiple treatment modalities unavailable to the primary-care practitioner. Patients must have pain controlled on a round-the-clock basis. Often this can be done with oral drugs, especially long-acting morphine derivatives.

Patients will have an anemia (normochromic) of chronic disease and hypoalbuminemia. Consultation with a nutritionist or a dietician experienced in the care of cachexia is necessary. If the patient has a deep jaundice, there may be malabsorption of the fat-soluble vitamins and diminished production of vitamin K-dependent clotting factors. Because of the malabsorption, steatorrhea, the hallmark of malabsorption, may be severe. The patient will probably be given pancreatic enzyme supplements, and should maintain a low-fat diet and abstain from alcohol (Beers & Berkow, 2000).

Elders who are candidates for surgery will often have postoperative delayed gastric emptying as a particularly distressing problem. This may resolve spontaneously over a period of time. Using prokinetic drugs such as metoclopromide may be useful (Lillemoe et al., 2000). Interestingly, erythromycin, also a prokinetic, has been shown to be effective for management.

Nursing diagnoses and plan of care. See description of previous cancers.

Diagnosis. Only biopsy reveals a certain diagnosis (ACS, 2002). However, when the patient with early presentation of jaundice appears, a high index of suspicion is warranted and ultrasound (US) or CT will confirm the obstruction of dilated intra- and extrahepatic bile ducts. CT is somewhat more specific and sensitive than US (90–95%) and will show a pancreatic mass and detect liver metastases or local vascular invasion (Lillemoe et al., 2000; Steer, 2002). ERCP (Endoscopic retrograde cholangiopancreatography) is used for patients whose diagnosis is not revealed by US or CT.

Labs will reveal an elevated serum bilirubin and alkaline phosphatase, and mild anemia. Tumor markers are elevated in advanced, incurable disease (Steer, 2002). The most widely used is serum concentration of cancer associated antigen 19-9 (CA 19-9). Its sensitivity and specificity are 80–90%.

Preoperative staging will occur to determine the feasibility of surgery and other therapies. If there are liver metastases, survival is very limited and conservative therapy is warranted to preserve quality of life.

Interventions, treatments, alternative therapy. All the therapeutic modalities are used to extend survival and to relieve symptoms. There is rarely a cure (ACS, 2002). For all stages of pancreatic cancer, the 1-year survival rate is only 21% and the 5-year rate is 5%.

Surgery. Surgical resection is the only potentially curative therapy for pancreatic cancer (Fernandez-del Castillo & Jimenez, 2002). However, because the disease presents so late in its course, only 15–20% of patients are candidates for surgery. The 5-year survival is 25–30% for node-negative survivors of pancreatectomy and 10% for node-positive tumors.

Radiation therapy. This is important therapy for elders with pancreatic cancer who are candidates for surgery. Nearly one-half of patients relapse after surgery with local or regional recurrence (Lillemoe et al., 2000) and radiation therapy will prolong life and provide some palliation of symptoms. Often RT is combined with chemotherapy.

Chemotherapy. Single agent gemcitabine is standard chemotherapy treatment for advanced pancreatic cancer (Hidalgo, 2001), although promising new regimens and novel agents are currently being investigated (ACS, 2002).

Other. Although androgen receptors have been found in pancreatic cancers, and testosterone seems to stimulate cancer growth, androgens and estrogens are still considerations for therapy. Trials with tamoxifen have shown little benefit at this time.

Palliation. Few patients are eligible for surgery and potential cure. Palliation of symptoms is needed to maximize quality of life. Surgery can be done but nonoperative palliation has fewer complications (Lillemoe et al., 2000). However, without surgery many patients will have recurrent jaundice and obstruction of the gastric outlet. Lillemoe states that surgical palliation offers the only chance for long-term palliation of the three major symptoms of pancreatic cancer: pain, duodenal obstruction, and obstructive jaundice. This means the patient would have a gastrojejunostomy. For pain, intraoperative injection of the celiac axis with 50% alcohol relieves subsequent pain.

Alternative therapy. No alternative therapies have been found to benefit elders with pancreatic cancer.

Health promotion and quality of life issues. Maintaining quality of life in these patients means constant follow-up. The disease can be very aggressive and cause profound problems to the patient and family. Regular oncology appointments and supportive care from others will be necessary. Management of depression is needed since the prognosis is so poor. Finding foods that will be of interest to the patient may be difficult for the family or caregiver and they need support throughout the remaining life of the patient.

Follow-up care. Malnourished patients are less able to tolerate surgery, radiation, chemotherapy, and the intense care that will be needed (Wilkes, 2000). Poor nutrition beckons infection, wounds, fistula formation, pneumonia, UTIs, pulmonary embolus, MI, and bowel obstruction. Any of these complications will diminish quality of life considerably and may require hospitalization.

Treatment side effects (chemotherapy, radiation, and surgery) can be serious. Recovery from surgery can take months in the healthiest individual. Anorexia is a common side effect of chemotherapy and RT, as is fever. There may be skin problems with RT.

Concurrent medical conditions need to be followed. Visits to the primary health caregiver (physician or nurse practitioner) are often cancelled due to fatigue, depression, pain, and difficulty coping with everyday life.

SUMMARY

This chapter has presented a wide range of information on gastrointestinal cancers. Health care research has just begun to unravel the complex causes of these types of cancers. Older adults usually present at their primary care provider's office with vague symptoms of distress. Once the diagnostic test results are available, gastrointestinal cancers are more often than not found at advanced stages of disease. While surgery, radiation, and chemotherapy are treatments that are advancing the length of survival for older adults diagnosed with gastrointestinal cancers, prognosis remains guarded.

Learning the risk factors that increase the likelihood of gastrointestinal cancers is a first step to prevention. Knowing the warning signs and symptoms is vital to extending the life expectancy once a diagnosis of cancer is made. Early detection is the best form of lengthening survival.

REFERENCES

American Cancer Society (2002). Cancer facts and figures. Atlanta: Author.

American Cancer Society (2002-b). Cancer prevention and early detection: Facts and figures. Atlanta: Author.

American Cancer Society (2002-c). New campaign says get tested for colon cancer. Retrieved from *www.cancer.org/eprise/main/docroot/NWS_2_1x_The_Polyp_Man_M*

American Cancer Society (2002-d). New DNA test aids in early detection of colon cancer. Retrieved from *www.cancer.org/eprise/main/docroot/NWS/content/NWS_1_1x_New_DNA_Test_Ai*

Agency for Healthcare Research and Quality (2001). Screening for colorectal cancer every 5 years reduces mortality at costs similar to other cancer screening procedures. January, No. 245, p. 12.

Balducci, L. (2002). Cancer. In R. J. Ham, P. D. Sloane, & G. A. Warshaw (Eds.), *Primary care geriatrics* (4th ed.). St. Louis: Mosby.

Beers, M. H., & Berkow, R. (2000). *The Merck Manual of Geriatrics*, 3rd ed. Whitehouse, NJ: Merck.

Boock, C. (2000). Health blurb: Shiitake mushrooms. Medical College of Wisconsin Physicians and Clinics. Retrieved from *Healthlink.mcw.edu/article/95264210-3.html*

Cancer.gov (2002). What you need to know about stomach cancer. Retrieved from *www.cancer.gov/cancer_information/doc*

CancerNet, 2002. Managing eating problems during treatment. Retrieved from *www.cancernet.gov/peb/eating_hints/index*

Fernandez, E. (2001). Oral contraceptives and colorectal cancer risk: A meta-analysis. *British Journal of Cancer*, May, 84, 722–727.

Fernandez-del-Castillo, C., & Jimenez, R. E. (2002). Risk factors for and molecular pathogenesis of pancreatic cancer. *UpToDate 10(1)*, 2002.

Fidias, P. (2001). Chemotherapy for advanced esophageal cancer. UpToDate 2001. Retrieved from *www.uptodate.com*

Fong, Y. (1999). Surgical therapy of hepatic colorectal metastasis. *CA Cancer Journal for Clinicians, 49(4)*, 231–255.

Harris, G. J. C. (2002). Factors affecting survival after palliative resection of colorectal carcinoma are identified. *Colorectal Disease 2002, 4(1)*, 31–5.

Healthandage (2002). Colorectal cancer. Retrieved from *www.healthandage.com/html/res/com/ConsConditions/CancerColorectalcc.html*

Hidalgo, M. (2001). GI Malignancies: Are We Changing the Standards of Care? 37th Annual Meeting of American Society of Clinical Oncology, May 14.

Jellin, J. M., Ed. (2002). Natural medicines, comprehensive database. Stockton, CA: Natural Database.

Jemel, A., Thomas, A., Murray, T., & Thun, M. (2002). Cancer statistics 2002. *CA Cancer Journal for Clinicians, 52(1)*, 23–45.

Lazcano-Ponce, E. C., Miquel, J. F., Munoz, N., Herrero, R., Ferrecio, C., Wistuba II, Alonso de Ruiz, P., Aristi Urista, G., & Nerri, F (2001). Epidemiology and molecular pathology of gallbladder cancer. *CA Cancer Journal for Clinicians, 51(6)*, 349–364.

Lillemoe, K. D., Yeo, C. J., & Cameron, J. L. (2000). Pancreatic cancer: State-of-the-art care. *CA Cancer Journal for Clinicians, 50(4)*, 241–268.

Lowe, R. C., Kim, R. D., Chari, R. S., & Afdhal, N. H. (2001). Epidemiology; pathogenesis; and classification of cholangiocarcinoma. UpToDate.

Macdonald, J. S. (2001). Fighting the Odds: Advances in Colorectal Cancer Diagnosis and Treatment. 37th Annual Meeting of the American Society of Clinical Oncology, May 14. Retrieved from *www.medscape.com/medscape/cno/2001/ASCOCME/Story.cfm?story_id=2223*

Matsumoto, S. (2002). Cimetidine can dramatically increase the survival of colorectal cancer patients. *British Journal of Cancer, 86,* 159–60, 161–67.

Mayer, R. J. (2000). Esophageal cancer. Retrieved from *www.harrisonsonline.com/server-java/Arknoid/amed/harrisons/do_chapt ers/ch090/ch*

MedicineNet-a (2002). Oral cancer. Retrieved from *www.focusoncancer.com*

MedicineNet-b (2002). Esophagus cancer. Retrieved from *www.focusoncancer.com/script/main/Art.asp*

MedicineNet-c (2002). Stomach cancer. Retrieved from *www.focusoncancer.com/script/main/Art*

MedicineNet-d (2002). Liver cancer. Retrieved from *www.focusoncancer.com/script/main/Art.asp?li=MNI&ArticleKey=1917&page=5*

Miller, B. A. (1996). Racial/ethnic patterns of cancer in the U.S. Bethesda, MD: National Cancer Institute.

Nair, S. (2002). Deaths from hepatocellular carcinoma have increased over the past 30 years in USA. *American Journal of Gastroenterology, 97*(1), 167–171.

National Cancer Institute (2001). A phase II trial of oral thalidomide as an adjuvant agent following metastasectomy in patients with recurrent colorectal cancer. Patient Recruitment and Public Liaison Office, 1-800-411-1222.

National Cancer Institute (2002). Mistletoe extracts. Retrieved from *www.cancer.gov/cancer_information/doc*

National Cancer Institute, National Center for Complementary and Alternative Medicine (2002). Questions and answers about Coenzyme Q10. Retrieved from *cis.nci.nih.gov/fact/9_16.htm*

National Institutes of Health (1998). Colonoscopy. NIH publication 98-4331. Retrieved from *www.niddk.nih.gov/health/digest/pubs/diagtest/colo.htm*

Novartis Foundation for Gerontology (2002). Further considerations: Cancer. Retrieved from *www.healthandage.com/html/res/primer/furthercon.htm*

Russell, R. M., & Mason, J. B. (2000). Preventing colon cancer: Does diet matter? Retrieved from *www.cyberounds.com/conferences/nutrition.html.9/28/2000*

Ryan, D. P. (2001). Clinical features, staging and treatment of anal cancer. UpToDate 9(3)01.

Sargent, D. J. (2001). Older patients with colon cancer benefit from chemotherapy. Retrieved from *www.cancer.gov/clinical_trials/doc.aspx?viewid=037f1039-bd11-4a46*

Savarese, D. M. F. (2001). Patient information: Treatment of rectal cancer. UpToDate 9(3) 01.

Schwartz, J. M., & Carithers, R. L. (2001). Epidemiology and etiologic associations of primary hepatocellular carcinoma. UpToDate 9(3)2001.

Schwartz, J. M., Stuart, K. E., & Carithers, R. L. (2001). Treatment of primary hepatocellular carcinoma. UpToDate 9(3)2001.

Sial, S. H., & Catalano, M. F. (2001). GI tract cancers in the elderly. *Gastroenterology Clinics of North America, 30*(2), 565–590.

Spencer, G. M. (2002). Laser therapy followed by brachytherapy for palliating advanced malignant dysphagia. *Gut, 50*(2), 224–227.

Steer, M. L. (2002). Clinical manifestations, diagnosis, and surgical staging of exocrine pancreatic cancer. UpToDate 10(1)2002.

Taguchi, A., et al. (2001). Selective postoperative inhibition of gastrointestinal opioid receptors. *New England Journal of Medicine, 345*(13), 935–940.

Weeks, J., & Nelson, H. (2002). Laparoscopic colon cancer surgery offers little QOL benefit. Journal of the American Medical Association. Retrieved January 16, 2002 from *www.cancer.gov/clinical_trials/doc.aspx?viewid=edaf3db0-69ad-4801*

Wilkes, G. (2000). Nutrition: The forgotten ingredient in cancer care. *AJN, 100*(4), 46–51.

Yamaji, Y. (2002). Weak response to H. pylori antibody is high risk for gastric cancer. *Scandanavian Journal of Gastroenterology, 37*, 148–153.

Zakko, W., & Zakko, S. F. (2002). Gallbladder polyps and cholesterolosis. UpToDate 10(1) 2002.

—9—

Nutrition and Gastrointestinal Diseases

Barbara Resnick

Due to normal age changes as well as life style (i.e., low-fiber diet, smoking, and alcohol use) and use of medications, older adults are at increased risk of developing gastrointestinal problems such as malignancies, ulcerations, and diverticular disease. There is often no cure for these gastrointestinal problems. Optimal management, however, can be achieved by modifying the older adult's diet.

COLON AND RECTAL CANCER

The prevention of colon and rectal cancer is an important focus of health promotion in older adults. Numerous dietary interventions have been tested including such things as maintaining optimal weight, eating more fruits and vegetables, getting sufficient calcium, increasing fiber intake, and limiting red meat or saturated fat intake. Current findings (Toyonaga, Okamatsu, Sasaki, Kimura, Saito, Shimizu, et al., 2000) suggest that consumption of fruits and vegetables cuts the risk of bowel and rectal cancer. The evidence for benefits from a higher-fiber diet is not conclusive. While fiber intake clearly helps decrease the incidence of constipation, it may not necessarily be good for preventing colorectal cancers.

ESOPHAGEAL CANCER

Rates of adenocarcinoma of the esophagus have increased six to eightfold since the 1970s, which is more rapidly than any other cancer in the United States. Moreover, the five year survival rate of this cancer is only 12%. The rise of esophageal cancer is believed to be due to reflux disease. Reflux is exacerbated by a diet that includes foods that contain caffeine, chocolate, alcohol, and high levels of fat. These foods all relax the sphincter between the stomach and the esophagus. One study (Mayne, Risch, Dubrow, Chow, Gammon, Vaughan, et al., 2001) noted that a plant-based diet actually decreased the risk of developing esophageal cancer. It was noted that fiber, vitamin C, folate, and beta-carotene protected individuals against developing esophageal cancer. Moreover, people who ate more animal products had a higher risk (Mayne, Risch, Dubrow, Chow, Gammon, Vaughan, et al., 2001). It is not clear, however, whether it is the meat, or the lack of fruits and vegetables in a meat-based diet, that increases the risk of esophageal cancer. The recommendations at this point in time suggest avoiding cigarettes and alcohol, maintaining appropriate body weight, and getting at least the recommended amount of fruits, vegetables, and whole grains.

GASTROESOPHAGEAL REFLUX DISEASE

Gastroesophageal reflux disease (GERD) includes the constellation of symptoms and consequences that occur due to esophageal reflux (see chapter 3). The nutritional implications of GERD must be considered in older adults as the discomfort associated with GERD can result in either weight loss or gain. Moreover, dietary interventions are an important aspect of disease management. While each older adult is different and responds differently to foods, general guidelines can be recommended. Moreover, older adults should be encouraged to eat small frequent meals rather than three large meals, to eat a diet high in protein, and to avoid reclining for several hours after eating.

There are certain foods that are known to increase gastric acid and those that directly damage the gastric mucosa. Alcohol both directly damages the gastric mucosa and stimulates gastric acid secretion, as does caffeine, garlic, paprika, horseradish, mustard, and other spices. Black pepper, chili powder, cloves, nutmeg, and mustard seed have been thought to cause some local irritation of the mucosa although this only occurs after consuming large amounts of these spices. Protein foods have a dual role related to gastric content and secretions. They act as a buffer but their buffering action is only temporary. Once the protein digestion products reach the antrum, they stimulate the secretion of gastrin and thus the secretion of gastric acid.

GASTROENTERITIS

Gastroenteritis is an inflammation of the gastric and mucous membrane and may be due to infection, either viral, bacterial, or protozoan. Foods and toxic agents in foods, as well as allergic or chemical reactions and enzyme deficiencies can also cause gastroenteritis. Dietary management is useful, in terms of both identification of the cause and treatment. A careful dietary history may help to identify contributors to gastroenteritis for any individual patient. Treatment should focus on fluid replacement, with consideration of electrolytes. Gatorade is one of the cheapest replacement options available. The BRATY diet continues to be recommended for dietary management once gastroenteritis has occurred (Table 9.1). This diet should be continued until diarrhea resolves.

CHOLELITHIASIS

Cholelithiasis refers to the formation of calculi or gallstones. The formation of gallstones puts the individual at risk of acute cholecystitis. Contributing

TABLE 9.1   BRATY Diet for Gastroenteritis

B:	Bananas
R:	Rice or rice cereal
A:	Apples, cooked
T:	Tea and toast
Y:	Yogurt, preferably with active cultures

*Bulking agents are also useful as a dietary supplement

(Resnick, 2002)

factors are regular intake of alcohol, and a high-fat, low-fiber diet. Consequently, treatment should focus on eating a low-fat, high-fiber diet. During acute attacks, however, clear fluids should be initiated and advanced as tolerated.

DIVERTICULOSIS/DIVERTICULITIS

Diverticulosis, the presence of colonic diverticula, occurs in two-thirds of the American population over the age of 60 (Stollman & Raskin, 1999). Diverticulosis is an outpouching in the colon at sites of insertion of the penetrating blood vessels. Diverticula are most common in the descending colon and sigmoid. Generally, there are no symptoms associated with diverticulosis until the bowel perforates; then there is infection or acute bleeding. When there is obstruction of the diverticula by stool and microperforation, diverticulitis occurs. At this point the older individual may complain of pain in the left lower quadrant, have a low-grade fever, elevated white count, and blood in the stool.

Treatment of acute diverticulitis includes a course of antibiotics and several days in which the bowel is allowed to rest and only clear liquids are given. Patients should be instructed to avoid foods that have small seeds, like tomatoes and berries, and increase the amount of soft bulk—like oats, apples, pears, and psyllium. Since low-fiber diets are associated with colonic diverticulosis, it is postulated that active therapy with higher-fiber diets might prevent diverticular disease. This theory of diverticular "prophylaxis" is supported by results from the Health Professionals Follow-Up Study, which prospectively followed 51,529 U.S. male health professionals (Aldoori et al., 1998). Although the results were fairly linear, suggesting increasing benefit with increasing fiber intake, the greatest benefit was seen in those individuals consuming an average of 32 g/day of total fiber (Table 9.2). Further analysis of this large epidemiological study also described a similar protective effect of physical activity on the development of symptomatic diverticulosis, and no effect was seen from alcohol, smoking, or caffeine consumption (Aldoori et al., 1995). Patients should be cautioned to gradually increase their fiber intake and maintain adequate hydration, to avoid transiently worsening their symptoms.

IRRITABLE BOWEL SYNDROME

Irritable bowel syndrome (IBS) is associated with the primary symptoms of alternating constipation and diarrhea. In addition, patients may have

TABLE 9.2   Fiber Content of Common Foods

Type of Food	Amount of Dietary Fiber per Average Serving
Cereals	(1/2 cup serving)
Fiber One	13 gm
Raisin Bran	3.0
All-Bran	8.4
Bran Flakes	7.8
Shredded Wheat	2.3
Vegetables	(1/2 cup serving)
Lettuce	1.0
Carrots	2.0
Celery	1.0
Cabbage	2.0
Broccoli	3.2
Brussels sprouts	2.3
Peas	6.0
Potatoes	3.0
Corn	2.6
Legumes	
Beans	8.5–10.0
Sunflower seeds	3.8
Sesame seeds	6.3
Walnuts	2.1
Peanuts	2.7
Almonds	2.6
Pecans	2.3
Fruit	
Bananas	1.5
Apples	2.0
Grapefruits	.6
Oranges	2.0
Peaches	2.0
Raspberries	4.6
Strawberries	1.6
Breads	(one slice)
English muffins	1.0
White bread	1.0
Whole wheat breads	1.3
Meats/Fish/Chicken/Cheese	0

Resnick, B. (2001). Constipation. In A. Adelman & M. Daley, *20 common problems in geriatrics*. New York: McGraw Hill.

lower left quadrant discomfort, distention, excessive flatus, and incomplete evacuation. Generally there is mucosal inflammation in the colon and/or small bowel that causes symptoms of bloody or nonbloody diarrhea and pain. There also may be nausea, vomiting, weight loss, and fever. Crohn's disease and ulcerative colitis are two common types of IBS. Crohn's disease is present when all the layers of the bowel wall are inflamed. In ulcerative colitis the inflammation is limited to the mucosa and submucosa, involves only the colon, and is usually continuous beginning in the rectum and involving any contiguous segment of the colon.

There is no cure for IBS. However the goal of treatment is to decrease intestinal and systemic inflammation as well as the patients' symptoms. For most people, diet goes a long way toward controlling IBS. A useful start to determine if symptoms are exacerbated by specific foods is to keep a "food symptoms" diary and record the time of day, the type of food eaten and the amount. General food guidelines are to eat *fewer* greasy, high-fat foods, avoid "gassy" foods like raw vegetables, apples with the peel, cabbage, cauliflower, dried peas, beans, nuts, and spicy or hot-flavored foods. High-fiber foods or supplements should be encouraged as tolerated (Table 9.2). Patients should be encouraged to drink water instead of caffeine, alcohol, or sugary drinks (they're intestinal stimulants). Diet management is very personal and individuals must learn what they can and cannot tolerate in terms of diet. A good starting point is to begin with a low-fiber diet including such foods as bread, applesauce, bananas, rice, and a psyllium supplement. This diet allows the body to adjust to a consistent source and amount of fiber.

NUTRITION OVERVIEW: CURRENT RECOMMENDATIONS

New recommendations for daily food intake have been developed for adults 70 years of age and older (Table 9.3). These guidelines recommend that fats, oils, and sweets be used sparingly, and the appropriate number of servings per food group be adhered to. In addition, eight 8-ounce servings of water are recommended.

ENERGY REQUIREMENTS

Generally speaking, older adults need the same nutrients, protein, carbohydrate, fat, vitamins, minerals, and water as younger individuals, but the

TABLE 9.3   Daily Requirements for Food Intake for the Elderly

- Bread group—six servings
- Vegetable group—three servings
- Fruit group—two servings
- Dairy group—two servings
- Meat group—two servings
- Fats/oils group—use sparingly

*A serving is $1/2$ cup; medium size fruit; 1 slice of bread; 3 ounces meat

(Resnick, 2002)

amounts needed could differ. As people age there is a tendency to become more sedentary and to use less energy (fewer calories) than they did in younger years. Moreover, with age the body uses energy at a slower rate. Although calorie needs vary depending on activity level, many older adults need about 1,600 calories daily. Chosen carefully, those 1,600 calories can be nutrient-packed and can supply the minimum recommendations from the "food pyramid." Depending on the individual, there may be concerns about weight loss or weight gain. It is helpful, therefore, to determine what the ideal body weight for the individual should be. Ideal body weight is easily determined by obtaining a height and weight chart and doing some simple calculations (Table 9.4). If an older individual is over 120% of his or her ideal body weight then it is likely they have metabolically inactive stores of fat.

It is also possible to calculate the total daily energy requirement (TDE) for the older adult, depending on his or her circumstance. Daily energy requirements decrease each year after age 35 and are calculated using the following: basal energy requirement, or the amount of energy required at

TABLE 9.4   Calculating Ideal Body Weight

For females: 100 pounds for the first five feet and add 5 pounds for each inch thereafter.

For males: 106 pounds for the first five feet and add 6 pounds for each inch thereafter.

Percent of ideal body weight: Actual body weight/ideal body weight

If older adults are over 120% of ideal body weight they are likely to have metabolically inactive stores of fat.

(Resnick, 2002)

complete rest to perform normal bodily functions, multiplied by a known activity factor and an injury factor (Table 9.5).

Protein

With regard to protein requirements, the current recommendations are that older adults need at least five ounces, or two servings, of protein a day. However, for some elderly people, protein-rich foods such as meat or poultry may be hard to chew. In addition, some may not buy meat, poultry, or fish because they can be more expensive than other foods. Table 9.6 provides some choices that can be recommended to facilitate an appropriate intake of protein.

TABLE 9.5   Calculating Total Daily Energy Requirements
(Basal energy requirement* × Activity Factor × Injury Factor = Total Daily Energy Requirement)

Activity Factor	Activity Factor/Injury Factor
Confined to bed	1.0–1.1
Out of bed	1.2–1.3
Normal activity (i.e., routine activities of daily living)	1.4–1.8
Extreme activity (i.e., beyond activities of daily living)	1.9–2.0
Surgery	1.1
Minor	
Major	1.2
Infection	1.2
Mild	
Moderate	1.4
Severe	1. 6
Trauma	
Skeletal	1.3
Head	1.6
Blunt	1.3
Burns	
40% body surface	1.5
100% body surface	1.9
Maintenance with no injury	1.0

Resnick, B. (2002)
*Basal Energy Expenditure = weight kcal + height kcal − age kcal (see Appendix?)

TABLE 9.6   Ways to Facilitate Protein Intake in Older Adults

Choose tender cuts of meat: chicken, turkey or ground meat
Have teeth, gums, and/or dentures checked regularly if chewing is a problem
Encourage use of soft dairy products: milk, cheese, and yogurt
Consider use of alternative proteins: soybean as found in tofu or tempeh
If money is an issue, stretch meat, poultry, and fish in casserole dishes or eat them in
   small portions
Consider less expensive protein sources such as eggs, beans, and peanut butter

(Resnick, 2002)

Calcium

With age there is an increased need for calcium. Moreover, calcium is not well absorbed in the older individual. To help maintain bone mass and reduce the risk of osteoporosis, calcium recommendations increase by 20% for older people (Abrams, 2001). Both men and women over age 50 should consume at least 1,200 milligrams of calcium each day. Men, however, should be careful not to exceed more than 2,000 mg per day of calcium as this has been linked to an increased risk of prostate cancer. Milk, cheese, and yogurt are the best sources of calcium. In addition, dark green leafy vegetables, fish with edible bones, tofu made with calcium sulfate, and calcium fortified fruit juices and cereal also have significant amounts of calcium. In addition many cereals, juices, and other foods are fortified with calcium. Conversely, in some individuals a high caffeine intake can increase calcium loss from the body (Miller, Jarvis, & McBean, 2001). These individuals have a loss in a gene that is involved in making vitamin D. Since it is impossible to know who those individuals are, it is recommended that older individuals keep caffeine intake to no more than 300 milligrams per day (two cups of brewed coffee, four cups of tea, or six cans of cola). Older adults may think that there is no benefit to increasing calcium intake at their age. These individuals may need to be convinced that it is never too late to benefit from increased calcium intake.

Vitamin D

Along with calcium it is essential to make sure that older adults get sufficient amounts of Vitamin D in their diets. Vitamin D helps deposit calcium in bones and helps protect against bone disease by keeping bones stronger (Patel, Collins, Bullock, Swaminathan, Blake, & Fogelman, 2001). Vitamin

D is known as the "sunshine vitamin" because the body makes it after sunlight, or ultraviolet light, hits the skin. Twenty to 30 minutes of sun exposure two to three times per week is adequate. However, for institutionalized or housebound older adults vitamin D can be obtained from foods. Sunscreen, however, blocks the ultraviolet rays that the skin needs to make vitamin D. In some states from late fall through early spring the sun's ultraviolet light is too weak to make vitamin D. Therefore, the easiest solution is to take an ordinary multivitamin with 600 IU of vitamin D. Most milk is fortified with vitamin D, as are cereals. You should check the nutrition facts panel to see if Vitamin D has been added.

Iron

Older adults do not generally need more iron-rich foods than younger individuals. Iron deficiency is a common problem and a common cause of anemia, but this is not often related to intake of iron. Rather, the loss of iron is more likely to be due to blood loss either from the gastrointestinal tract or some other site. When iron levels are low iron supplementation should be given. To facilitate the absorption of iron it can be given with Vitamin C. For older adults who do not tolerate iron supplements, foods rich in iron should be recommended (Table 9.7).

Along with iron, when there are concerns about anemia, folate and B_{12} must also be considered. Folate helps the body make red blood cells and can lead to anemia if intake is low. Good sources include leafy green vegetables, fruits, beans, enriched grain products, wheat germ, and some fortified cereals. Vitamin B_{12} works with folate to make red blood cells. Too little vitamin B_{12} can also lead to anemia, and in some older adults is linked to neurological problems. Meat, poultry, fish, eggs, and dairy foods are all good sources of vitamin B_{12}.

Vitamin K

Vitamin K helps blood clot as it is required for the synthesis of clotting factors II, VII, IX, and X in the liver. In the Framingham Osteoporosis

TABLE 9.7   Foods Rich in Iron

Choose iron-enriched cereals, beans, whole-grains, lean meat, and poultry
Enjoy a vitamin C-rich fruit or fruit juice at meals
Add a little meat, poultry, fish or beans to pasta or rice dishes

(Resnick, 2002)

Study, however, it was found that the higher the intake of vitamin K the higher the bone density (Hannan, Felson, Dawson-Hughes, Tucker, Cupples, Wilson, et al., 2000). It is not clear how much vitamin K is enough, but in the Framingham study, those at highest risk got an average of 60 micrograms a day and those at the lowest risk averaged 250 micrograms a day. Current research continues to explore the relationship between vitamin K and bone health. In the meantime, it is recommended that women consume at least 90 micrograms of vitamin K daily and that men consume 120 micrograms. This can be done easily by eating salads and greens such as collards, spinach, brussel sprouts, romaine lettuce, or broccoli (1/2 cup portions), or Viactiv Soft Calcium chews which have about half of the daily requirement per chew. For older adults who take Coumadin it is important to record dosing of the vitamin K and monitor the Prothrombin time and International Ratio and dose the Coumadin accordingly.

Antioxidants

Antioxidants such as vitamin C, E, selenium, and carotenoids do not for certain prevent the development of chronic disease, or help limit the gradual build-up of cellular damage as hypothesized (National Academy of Sciences, 2000). Ongoing research, however, continues to explore this question. In the meantime, the National Academy of Sciences has set Tolerable Upper Intake Levels (ULs) to help guide those individuals who would like to continue to take them as preventatives.

Vitamin C dosages were based on side effects of diarrhea at higher dosages. There have been some additional, unfounded reports about vitamin C in large dosages clogging arteries, but those studies were not scientifically sound, and larger epidemiological studies had no such findings (Zhang, Giovannucci, Hunter, Rimm, Ascherio, Colditz, et al., 2001). There is no conclusive data as to whether vitamin C increases the risk of cancer or decreases cancer treatment as previously hypothesized. The new Recommended Dietary Allowances (RDAs) set by the NAS is 75 mg for a women and 90 mg for a man, with a daily value of 60 mg and a UL of 2,000 mg.

Vitamin E, which is a fat-soluble vitamin, was noted to possibly cause hemorrhages in humans as this was the result when high doses were given to rats. These findings have not been well supported in large studies (Jacobs, Connell, McCullough, Chao, Jonas, Rodriguez, et al., 2002). High dosages of vitamin E may cause bleeding in individuals who are deficient in vitamin K, or in those who are taking anticoagulants such as Coumadin. Vitamin K and vitamin E may also compete for absorption in the gut and vitamin

E may decrease the absorption of K causing the bleeding. As with vitamin K, those taking vitamin E that are also on Coumadin should have PT and INR levels closely monitored. The new RDA for vitamin E is 22 IU of the natural (d-alpha tocopherol) and 33 IU of the synthetic (dl-alpha tocopherol), and 1,500 IU upper level for the natural and 1,100 IU is the upper limit for the synthetic.

Selenium

Upper limits have also been established for those interested in taking selenium supplements. The upper limits of selenium were based on the side effect of lost or brittle hair or nails. Other possible signs of toxicity from selenium include gastrointestinal disturbances, fatigue, and nervous system abnormalities (Mayne, Risch, Dubrow, Chow, Gammon, Vaughan, et al., 2001). Unfortunately, it is difficult to determine the need to supplement as the levels of selenium in foods vary based on the region. Some preliminary studies have shown that selenium supplementation may lower the risk of cancer, but these findings are only preliminary (Mayne, Risch, Dubrow, Chow, Gammon, Vaughan, et al., 2001). Ongoing research will continue to explore this. In the meantime the daily recommendation for selenium is 55 micrograms, with no specific daily value set, but an upper limit of 400 micrograms.

Carotenoids have no ULs established. Carotenoids have been associated with lung health and decreased risk of cancer (Schunemann, McCann, Grant, Trevisan, Muti, & Freudenheim, 2002), although these findings are not conclusive. Beta-carotene, the most widely known carotenoid, is converted into vitamin A in the body. Older adults should be encouraged to eat foods rich in beta-carotene such as carrots, cantaloupe, and sweet potatoes.

Fluid Intake

Older adults require the same amount of fluid as other adults, i.e., 1800 to 2500 cc/day of water. This is necessary for urinary excretion and to replace losses from insensible perspiration. Additional fluids should be added to replace water lost by excessive sweating, vomiting, diarrhea, or tube drainage. Deficient water intake can result in dehydration. For numerous reasons, older adults are particularly at risk for dehydration (Table

9.8). These individuals should be encouraged to take at least eight to twelve cups of fluid per day. Food provides some water, but drinking at least eight cups of water daily is advised. Water can come from all kinds of beverages, including juice, milk, soup, tea, coffee, and soft drinks. Plain water is great, too. Remember that juice, milk, and soup provide other nutrients as well.

ASSESSMENT OF NUTRITIONAL STATE

History

In order to evaluate the nutritional status of older adults it is helpful to evaluate risk factors (Table 9.9) for malnutrition and do a nutritional history (Table 9.10). In addition, if possible, the older individual should be encouraged to complete the Nutritional Assessment to further help identify potential risk factors for malnutrition (Table 9.11).

Physical Exam

Physical findings can also be used to identify older individuals with nutritional impairment (Table 9.12). Weight is generally the best marker of

TABLE 9.8   Risk Factors for Dehydration

Decreased thirst perception
Decreased ability to concentrate urine
Decreased renin activity and aldosterone secretion
Functional impairment resulting in difficulty obtaining and consuming fluids
Cognitive impairment resulting in difficulty remember how to drink and when to drink
Medications (i.e., diuretics and laxatives)
Fever
Diarrhea or vomiting
Draining wounds
Excessive sweating
Increased respiratory rate
Bleeding
Use of specialty beds

(Resnick, 2002)

TABLE 9.9   Risk Factors for Malnutrition

Risk Indicator	Indicative Signs and Symptoms
Weight loss	Weight loss of > 5% body weight in 1 month Weight loss of > 7.5% body weight in 3 months Weight loss of > 10% body weight in 6 months Weight loss of > 20% body weight in 12 months
Change in appetite	Poor appetite with decreased food intake Change in taste Inability to keep food down
Change in bowel pattern	New onset constipation Persistent diarrhea
Change in cognition	Acute change with delirium indicative of acute illness Chronic progressive changes that may influence food intake and ability to eat
Difficulty swallowing or chewing	Coughing when attempting to swallow Recurrent pneumonias
Change in function	Decline in ability to perform activities of daily living which can influence ability to prepare and consume food
Fall	Underlying signs and symptoms of an acute respiratory or urinary infection or other acute illness
Loss of social support	Death of spouse, family member or change in living situation that may result in increased isolation or need to prepare food and eat alone
Loss of economic resources	Income of < $6,000 per year of spending or less than $30 a week for food Use of public assistance for food, shelter, or utilities

(Resnick, 2002)

TABLE 9.10 History for Nutritional Status

Focus Area	Additional Information
Chief complaint	Focus on history of weight loss to include weights over the past year; daily intake and ability to buy, prepare, and eat meals as appropriate. Explore for underlying signs and symptoms of illness.
Medical History	In particular explore for a history of: Alcoholism Arthritis Gastritis B_{12}or folate deficiency Bowel habit changes Cancer Cardiovascular disease Chronic pain Renal disease Chronic respiratory conditions Delirium Cognitive impairment Depression Diabetes Osteoporosis Thyroid disease Irritable bowel disease Diverticulitis/diverticulosis Recent acute illnesses
Medications	Cardiovascular drugs: diuretics, betablockers, procainamide, central alpha inhibitors Hypoglycemics/insulin Antiseizure medications Psychotropics: benzodiazepines, neuroleptics, selective serotonin receptor inhibitors, tricyclic antidepressants, Thyroid replacement Painkillers: nonsteroidal anti-inflammatory drugs or narcotics Total number of prescription drugs: > 6
Psychiatric history	Depression treatment and management Cognitive impairment treatment and management
Falls and fractures	History of events with focus on recent falls and fractures
Personal Health Habits	Alcohol intake Nicotine use Activity Dietary restrictions: i.e., low cholesterol, low sodium

(Resnick, 2002)

TABLE 9.11   Patient Nutritional Screening

I (or someone close to me) have/has an illness or condition that has caused me to change the amount and/or kind of food I eat.
I eat fewer than 2 meals per day.
I eat few fruits or vegetables a day.
I eat or drink few milk products(i.e., milk, yogurt, cheese) a day.
I drink less than 5 cups (8 oz. per cup) of fluid a day (i.e., water, juice, tea).
I have 3 or more drinks of beer, wine, or liquor almost everyday.
I have tooth or mouth problems that make it hard for me to eat.
I don't always have enough money to buy the food I need.
I eat alone most of the time.
I take 3 or more different prescribed or over-the-counter drugs a day.
Without wanting to, I have lost or gained 10 pounds in the last 6 months.
I am not always physically able to shop, cook, and/or feed myself.

0–2 YES	Good! Recheck your nutritional score in 6 months.
3–5 YES	**You are at moderate nutritional risk.** See what can be done to improve your eating habits and lifestyles. Your office on aging, senior nutrition program, senior citizens center, or health department can help.
6 or more YES	**You are at high nutritional risk.** Bring this checklist the next time you see your doctor, dietitian, or other qualified health or social service professional. Talk with them about any problems you may have. Ask for help to improve your nutritional health.

American Academy of Family Physicians Nutrition Screening Initiative (http://www.aafp.org/nsi/)

nutritional status. Weight should be obtained using the same scale, at the same time of the day. If the individual is in an institutional setting, it is useful to weigh him or her every week for four weeks to establish a baseline, and then every month thereafter to monitor for variance (AMDA, 2001).

In addition to weight, height should be obtained so that body mass index can be accurately calculated. For older adults who cannot stand upright to measure height, an approximation can be obtained by measuring arm span. Arm span measurements are done by measuring from fingertip to fingertip with the arms fully extended, or double the distance from extended fingertip to mid-sternum (Niedert, 1998). Another option is to measure knee height. Knee height is the distance from heel to knee, with the foot and knee at 90 degrees (Chumlea & Guo, 1992). Lastly, recumbent

TABLE 9.12   Physical Examination for Malnutrition

Focus Area	Assessment
Anthropometrics	Body mass index (BMI) which is the [weight in kilograms plus height in centimeters squared × 10,000] < 24 or 80% of the ideal body weight.
	Lean muscle mass decrease noted by mid-arm muscle mass below 10%
Laboratory findings	Triceps skin fold below 10% Serum albumin < 3.5
	Thyroxine binding prealbumin <10 mg/dl = severe risk; 10 to 17 mg/dl is a moderate risk
	Hemoglobin of < 12 grams/dl
	Cholesterol < 160 mg/dl
Physical Exam	Lymphocytes < 1,500/cm^3 Muscle wasting and weakness
	Peripheral neuropathy
	Xerostomia, cheilosis, angular fissures, glossitis, red beefy tongue, swollen or bleeding gums, dental loss and decay and infection, poor fitting dentures
	Swallowing difficulties particularly coughing after swallowing liquids or vomiting associated with eating
	Evidence of wound development or poor wound healing
	Vision or hearing changes
	Thyroid enlargement
Functional Assessment	Dependent edema Demonstration of ability to perform activities of daily living including bathing, dressing, eating, transferring, toileting, ambulation, and stair climbing, as appropriate
Cognitive and Mood Assessment	Testing to indicate cognitive ability using the Folstein Mini Mental State Exam (Folstein, Folstein, & McHugh, 1975)
	Testing to screen for depression using the Geriatric Depression Scale (Hoyle et al., 1999).

(Resnick, 2002)

height can be obtained by using a flexible tape and measuring the older adult when lying down. This measurement is approximately 1.5 inches greater than the standing height (Gray, Crider, Kelley, & Dickinson, 1985).

Once height and weight have been obtained it is possible to calculate the body mass index (BMI) using the following formula:

BMI = weight (kilograms)/height (in meters, squared) or [weight in pounds/ height in inches, squared] × 704.

A BMI between 23 and 25 is considered desirable. A BMI in the range of 25 to 30 is overweight, and over 30 is considered obese. A BMI between 19 and 23 is considered underweight and a BMI of less than 19 is considered severely underweight.

Oral Examination

A nutrition related evaluation of the mouth and lips is essential when evaluating nutritional status. In particular individuals should be evaluated for evidence of cheilosis or inflammation of the lips and associated angular stomatitis, or redness and breakdown in the corners of the mouth. This is commonly found in deficiencies of the B-complex vitamins. B-complex deficiency can also result in glossitis, or inflammation of the tongue. Sublingual redness of the tongue and increased vascularization is associated with a vitamin C deficiency. Secretions in the mouth, and evidence of dryness should also be considered as extreme dryness alters taste and makes eating difficult. Likewise teeth, gums, and dentures should be evaluated for fit and utility. A bedside swallowing evaluation should also be done (see chapter 2). This will help establish the older adult's ability to swallow comfortably and safely and consume a sufficient amount of nutrients.

Dermatologic Examination

Evidence of subcutaneous fat loss and of dryness of the skin should be identified. Floppy, loose skin and striae are consistent with weight loss in older adults. Nonspecific lesions, purpura and easy bruising, poorly healing wounds, and ulcers are also indicators of poor nutritional status. Edema of the skin in areas that are not dependent may be due to hypoproteinemia.

Musculoskeletal Examination

Muscular strength and mass can be indicators of poor nutritional status or of other muscular wasting diseases. The range and strength of movement of the upper extremities, including fine hand movements, are of significance in the preparation and consumption of food. Bone tenderness, especially over the vertebrae may be indicative of bone disease or fracture and consideration should be given as to whether or not there is evidence of osteopenia or osteoporosis. Appropriate interventions would be to at least explore the use of calcium and vitamin D. Impaired mobility also may be due to poor nutritional status, and may further exacerbate nutritional state by making it difficult to buy and prepare food and eat.

Gastrointestinal Examination

Evaluation of the gastrointestinal system with regard to evidence of pain, bleeding, obstruction, or irritation anywhere along the gastrointestinal system is important. Gastrointestinal pain associated with eating can certainly impact nutritional status. When gastrointestinal problems are identified, further exploration of the underlying cause of the problem should be done as long as the individual or the person holding power of attorney is willing to pursue this. Ultimately, the goal should be to identify the underlying cause of the symptoms and thereby improve nutritional status once the underlying problem is resolved.

Cognitive State

When evaluating older adults it is very useful to establish baseline cognitive ability and monitor this with any change in health status, medication regimen, living situation, or schedule. There are numerous tools that can be used to evaluate cognition including the Mini Mental State Exam (Folstein, Folstein, & McHugh, 1975) and the Clock Drawing Test (Watson, Arfken, & Birge, 1993). Testing using these types of tools allows the health care provider to follow cognitive changes over time and determine if they are acute (which would be indicative of a delirium) or chronic (indicating dementia). Regardless of the cause of the cognitive impairment, memory problems can result in the inability to buy food and prepare meals, and ultimately to the inability to remember how to chew and swallow food.

LABORATORY ASSESSMENTS ASSOCIATED
WITH NUTRITIONAL STATUS

The complete blood count (CBC) helps to indicate if the individual has an underlying anemia. Further testing including a B_{12} and folate, iron studies, and a reticulocyte count will help to establish the underlying cause of the anemia, and establish if it is due to nutritional intake. Serum B_{12} is not an indicator of generic poor nutritional status, but rather focuses on a lack of sufficient B_{12} in the system due to either intake or loss. Testing for folate, however, is a more appropriate indicator of poor nutritional status (see chapter 7).

A total lymphocyte count can be used directly as a measure of nutritional impairment. The lymphocyte counts give the clinician a sense of how functional the older adult's immune system is. A total lymphocyte count of less than 1500 per microliter may be regarded as abnormal, with a level of 1200 to 1500 per microliter being mildly impaired, 900 to 1200 being moderately impaired, and less than 900 indicative of severe nutritional impairment. Cholesterol levels are another useful indicator of poor nutritional status. A cholesterol level below 160 mg/100 ml would likely be associated with increased mortality. Likewise thyroid function can directly influence nutritional status (i.e., if the older adult has a hyper- or hypoactive thyroid).

The most commonly used laboratory screening of nutritional status has been the testing of albumin, transferrin, and prealbumin. Albumin, with its 17 to 21 day half-life, is sensitive to changes in nutritional status, slowly returning to normal levels when the nutritional deficiency is corrected. It is not, however, a good indicator of early malnutrition because of its long half-life. In addition, many disease states such as congestive heart failure, acute inflammatory process, liver disease, or trauma modify the level of albumin. Levels of albumin may be falsely high in individuals who are dehydrated, a common problem in older adults, and falsely low in older adults with any type of edema. Transferrin has a shorter half-life of eight to ten days, and therefore responds more quickly to deficiency and repletion. Transferrin, however, increases when there is iron deficiency, and is reduced in the face of chronic infections. The last of the three proteins commonly tested is prealbumin, also called transthyretin and thyroxine-binding prealbumin. The half-life of prealbumin is even shorter than that of transferrin, just two to three days, so that it is more sensitive to changes. Prealbumin levels are not greatly affected by mild renal or liver disease or edema. Prealbumin levels are, however, affected by hepatobiliary disease, inflammation, malignancy, and protein-wasting diseases of the intestines or kidneys. Both transferrin and prealbumin are more costly tests to run than albumin, and as such are not routinely included.

The total leukocyte count has also been used in the assessment of visceral protein stores. The total leukocyte count, which is normally 4,500 to

11,000/mm³, provides information about the immunological status of the patient. The immunologic defect is primarily a T-cell immunodeficiency. Levels less than 1,500/mm³ suggest immunodeficiency and impaired nutritional status.

Electrolyte changes may be indicative of nutritional problems. Hypernatremia, a higher than normal level of sodium in the blood, may be indicative of dehydration. Hyponatremia, on the other hand, may occur in individuals who severely restrict their sodium intake, although it is more commonly associated with medications as is hypokalemia.

LONG-TERM CARE NUTRITIONAL ASSESSMENT

For older adults in the long-term care setting the Minimum Data Set (MDS) is completed on admission to the facility and at intervals thereafter. Certain items in the MDS relate to nutritional status and risk factors for impaired nutritional state (Table 9.13). These items can be extracted from the computerized data base developed in each facility.

Malnutrition: Incidence and Risk

In the United States, the prevalence of malnutrition in the elderly is less than 1% in individuals who are independent and healthy. Estimates for other groups are 25% in the general population of elderly, 23% to 85% in nursing home residents, and 33% to 55% in those hospitalized (Thomas, Ashmen, Morley, & Evans, 2000). Noninstitutionalized persons age 65 and older are at increased risk for malnutrition because of poverty, social

TABLE 9.13   Minimum Data Set Indicators for Impaired Nutritional State

G1h	Inability to feed oneself
K1a	Chewing problems
K1b	Swallowing problems
K3a	Significant weight loss
K4a	Presence of taste alterations
K4c	Leaves 25% of food at most meals
K5d	Needs to use a syringe to facilitate intake
K5e	Therapeutic diets

(Resnick, 2002)

isolation, meal skipping, and the use of multiple prescription and nonprescription drugs (Cope, 1996). Malnutrition may develop or worsen during periods of acute stress, illness, trauma, or surgery (Dudek, 2000).

Malnutrition contributes to a progressive decline in health and places older adults at increased risk for complications such as weakness, delirium, or a fall (Thomas, Ashmen, Morley, & Evans, 2000). Moreover, for older adults who are acutely ill and hospitalized, there is a significant increased risk of morbidity (Dudek, 2000) and an indirect increase in costs due to prolonged recovery and stress (Schultz & Beach, 1999).

Causes of Malnutrition

Certain physical and mental problems can result in decreased intake of food and malnutrition, specifically depression, anxiety, diabetes, cancer, acute and chronic pain, and neurological problems including Parkinson's disease, stroke, and any type of cognitive impairment. Oral problems, a common finding in older adults, likewise can decrease food intake. Moreover, if the individual is only able to eat blenderized food there may be a decrease in the actual caloric intact when these foods are made with the addition of water.

Medications are another major cause of anorexia, and can result in decreased food intake and malnutrition. Drugs with anorexic effects include antidepressants, selective serotonin reuptake inhibitors, dopamine agonists, xanthine drugs, diuretiecs and hypertensive agents, and pain medication (i.e., opiates).

Treatment of Impaired Nutrition

In older adults poor health and poor nutrition often interact in a vicious circle: inadequate food intake promotes illness, and illness diminishes food intake. A number of scientific studies (Gloth, Tobin, Smith, & Meyer, 1996) have made clear that improving nutrition can contribute to improvements in both health and functioning in older adults. However, the decision to treat a malnourished patient must be based on what the patient or person holding power of attorney wants. Careful communication of the risks and benefits associated with an intervention is essential. Malnutrition, for example, often occurs at the end of life and instituting aggressive interventions may not actually improve the quality of life.

Decreasing the Risks of Impaired Nutrition

Treatment of impaired nutrition should be considered as an intervention that offers a reasonable expectation of benefit for the older individual. All of the factors identified as potential risk factors in the individual should be addressed. For example, if depression is recognized, treatment should be instituted whether this is medical management, the use of psychotherapy, or exercise. Medications that can be eliminated, particularly those that are known to alter taste or cause nausea, should be stopped or decreased.

Changes in the individual's eating environment should likewise be considered. Particularly for institutionalized older adults, the room in which meals are served should be pleasant and conducive to eating. Foods should be served in an attractive way. Encourage group dining and socialization around meals to facilitate intake. It may be particularly useful to encourage a predinner social hour in which small amounts of alcohol are served to increase appetite and encourage further food intake.

Attempts should be made in the home and institutional setting to serve preferred foods and culturally relevant meals. In the institutional setting invite families to bring in favorite foods and encourage the patient to eat these foods at times that are consistent with his or her wants. Meals, and the timing of meals, can certainly deviate from the tradition three times per day. Older adults ideally should be encouraged to eat smaller meals at more frequent intervals, i.e., every three hours if possible. Meals and snacks should be in a form that is easy for the individual to consume, for example, pureed or soft such as oatmeal, ice cream, yogurt, or mashed potatoes.

For older adults who are malnourished, all dietary restrictions should be liberalized. Any benefit in long-term disease management is not worth the risk of impaired nutritional state. With renal disease, however, there is some research to support that a protein restricted diet may delay the onset of dialysis (Fouque, Want, Laville, Boissel, & Cochrane Renal Group, 2000).

Diets of altered consistency, albeit for the safety of the older individual, are often unpalatable and visually unappealing. Older adults may reject them entirely. It is important to attempt to liberalize the diet as much as possible, and discuss the risk and benefits of doing so with the patient and/or person holding a health care power of attorney. Helping individuals to identify foods that are of the appropriate consistency for them to consume easily is also useful. Increasing the list of preferences, by informing the individual of different types of soft cheeses, puddings, soups, or casseroles that are soft and easily consumed, is useful.

Appetite Stimulants

The use of appetite stimulants should be considered on an individual basis. Exercise is one of the best nonpharmacologic approaches to appetite stimulation. Encouraging 30 minutes of exercise daily can potentially increase appetite overall. Examples of common pharmacologic interventions to increase appetite are shown in Table 9.14. These drugs may increase appetite or relieve nausea so caloric intake can be increased. However, the weight gained may consist of fat mass rather than lean body mass and patients may not regain strength even though they eat more (Oster, Enders, & Samuels, 1994). A newer group of drugs, the anabolic agents, work to increase body weight by promoting lean body mass through protein synthesis, or anabolism. Some anabolic agents are synthetic derivatives of testosterone. Essentially these drugs promote gains in muscle mass by increasing protein synthesis. The androgenic effects, however, are similar to those of male sex hormones. The effectiveness of these agents varies, and they should be initiated on a trial basis and evaluated at intervals. Some agents, such as megesterol acetate, will not be effective for at least two months. If the older individual gains weight and tolerates the treatment, the drugs should be continued for at least 12 weeks.

TABLE 9.14   Pharmacological Interventions to Stimulate Appetite

Drug Group	Common Associated Risks
Orexigenic Agents –Megestrol acetate (Megace) –Dronabinol (Marinol)	Phlebitis Pulmonary embolism Vaginal bleeding
Antidepressants –Remeron –Zoloft	Change in behavior Increased risk of seizure
Steroids –Dexamethason (Decadron, Hexadrol)	Muscle weakness Impaired wound healing Phleblitis and blood clots Infection Thinning of skin Decreased bone density
Anabolic Steroids –Oxandrolone (Oxandrin)	Virilizing side effects Alter liver function

(Resnick, 2002)

Supplemental Feedings

Dietary supplementation is commonly initiated in response to impaired nutritional states in older adults. Certainly this intervention is low risk for the individual. The goal of dietary supplements is to provide adequate energy and protein intake. Foods high in calories such as ice cream and pudding are ideal. In the event that the patient cannot consume adequate calories or is unwilling to eat sufficient quantities, the diet can be supplemented with any variety of products in the market specifically developed for this purpose.

Tube Feedings

Tube feedings either by nasogastric tubes or gastrointestinal tubes are another option for nutritional supplementation. Careful consideration must be given to the risks and benefits of starting tube feedings in older adults. Moreover, this decision needs to be made in conjunction with the patient and his or her health care power of attorney as appropriate. End-of-life care preferences and decisions related to tube feedings and supplement hydration should be initiated when doing initial assessments of the individual older adult. This discussion should be repeated, however, at yearly intervals since decisions about end-of-life care preferences may change over time (Nahm & Resnick, 2000). Health care providers should inform patients and appropriate care givers of the current state of knowledge related to nutrition at the end-of-life. Specifically, patients need to understand that they will not experience hunger at the end of life and may be satisfied with small amounts of food or liquids. Moreover, tube feedings do not ensure that the patient will be more comfortable or experience less suffering. Often tube feedings can cause diarrhea, abdominal pain, and local complications and irritation, as well as increase the risk of aspiration (Finucane, Chrismas, & Travis, 1999). Use of tube feeding may be appropriate when the older adult chokes during eating, when difficulty swallowing prevents oral intake of adequate calories, when there are head and neck surgeries or injuries that make eating impossible, and when there is a discontinuous gastrointestinal tract.

Tube feedings should initially be started at half-strength, 25cc per hour. The strength of the feedings can then be increased by one-quarter every four hours. Once at full strength the rate can be increased by 10cc every four hours until the goal rate is achieved. Residuals and tolerance of the patient should be closely monitored.

CONCLUSION

Nutritional status is an important aspect of care of the older adult, particularly those with abdominal problems. Any change in weight can have negative clinical consequences with regard to recovery from an acute event. In addition, it is possible that nutrition may have an impact on the development of abdominal diseases such as gastrointestinal malignancies. Careful assessment of nutritional status through history taking and physical examination, and education and guidance with regard to appropriate food intake, can help older adults maintain their highest level of health and well-being.

REFERENCES

Abrams, S. A. (2001). Calcium turnover and nutrition through the life cycle. *Proctology and Nutrition Society, 60*(2), 283–289.

Aldoori, W. H., Giovannucci, E. L., Rockett, H. R. H., et al. (1998). A prospective study of dietary fiber types and symptomatic diverticular disease in men. *Journal of Nutrition, 128,* 714–719.

Aldoori, W. H., Giovannucci, E. L., Rimm, E. B., et al. (1995). Prospective study of physical activity and the risk of symptomatic diverticular disease in men. *Gut, 36,* 276–282.

AMDA (2001). Clinical guideline for altered nutrition status. Columbia, MD: Author.

Chumlea, W. C., & Guo, S. (1992). Equations for predicting stature in white and black individuals. *Journal of Gerontology Medical Sciences, 47,* M197–M203.

Cope, K. (1996). Malnutrition in the elderly, a national crisis: Contributes to disease, illness, disability, death, escalates health care costs, decreases quality of life. Region X, U.S. Administration on Aging. Publication No. 017-062-00147-2. Washington, DC: U.S. Government Printing Office.

Dudek, S. G. (2000). Malnutrition in hospitals: Who's assessing what patients eat? *American Journal of Nursing, 100*(4), 36–42.

Finucane, T. E., Chrismas, C., & Travis, K. (1999). Tube feeding in patients with advanced dementia: A review of the evidence. *Journal of the American Medical Association, 282,* 1365.

Folstein, M., Folstein, S., & McHugh, P. (1975). Mini-mental state: A practical method for grading the cognitive state of patients for the clinician. *Journal of Psychiatric Research, 12,* 189–198.

Fouque, C., Want, P., Laville, M., Boissel, J., & Cochrane Renal Group (2000). Low protein diets delay end stage renal disease in non diabetic adults with chronic renal failure. Cochrane Database of Systematic Reviews. Retrieved from *http://www.update-software.com/cochrane/cochrane-frame.html.*).

Gloth, F. M. 3rd, Tobin, J. D., Smith, C. E., & Meyer, J. N. (1996). Nutrient intakes in a frail homebound elderly population in the community versus a nursing home. *Journal of the American Dietetic Association, 96*(6), 605–607.

Gray, D., Crider, J., Kelley, C., & Dickinson, L. (1985). Accuracy of recumbent height measurement. *Journal of Parenteral Enteral Nutrition, 9,* 712–715.

Hannan, M. T., Felson, D. T., Dawson-Hughes, B., Tucker, K. L., Cupples, L. A., Wilson, P. W., & Kiel, D. P. (2000). Risk factors for longitudinal bone loss in elderly men and women: The Framingham Osteoporosis Study. *Journal of Bone Mineral Research, 15*(4), 710–720.

Jacobs, E. J., Connell, C. J., McCullough, M. L., Chao, A., Jonas, C. R., Rodriguez, C., Calle, E. E., & Thun, M. J. (2002). Vitamin C, vitamin E, and multivitamin supplement use and stomach cancer mortality in the Cancer Prevention Study II cohort. *Cancer Epidemiologic Biomarkers Prevention, 11*(1), 35–41.

Mayne, S. T., Risch, H. A., Dubrow, R., Chow, W. H., Gammon, M. D., Vaughan, T. L., Farrow, D. C., Schoenberg, J. B., Stanford, J. L., Ahsan, H., West, A. B., Rotterdam, H., Blot, W. J., & Fraumeni, J. F. Jr. (2001). Nutrient intake and risk of subtypes of esophageal and gastric cancer. *Cancer Epidemiologic Biomarkers Prevention, 10*(10), 1055–1062.

Miller, G. D., Jarvis, J. K., & McBean, L. D. (2001). The importance of meeting calcium needs with foods. *Journal of the American College of Nutrition, 20*(2 Suppl.), 168S–185S.

Nahm, E., & Resnick, B. (2001). End of life care preferences of older adults. *Nursing Ethics, 8*(4), 532–543.

National Academy of Sciences (2000). Dietary reference intakes for vitamin C, E, selenium and carotenoids. National Academy. Proceedings of National Academy of Sciences, USA.

Niedert, K. (Ed.) (1998). *Nutrition care of the older adult.* Chicago: American Dietetic Association.

Oster, M., Enders, S., & Samuels, S. (1994). Megestrol acetate in patient with AIDS and cachexia. *Annals of Internal Medicine, 121,* 400–408.

Patel, R., Collins, D., Bullock, S., Swaminathan, R., Blake, G. M., & Fogelman, I. (2001). The effect of season and vitamin D supplementation on bone mineral density in healthy women: A double-masked crossover study. *Osteoporosis International, 12*(4), 319–325.

Resnick, B. (2001). Constipation. In A. Adelman & M. Daley, *20 common problems in geriatrics.* New York: McGraw Hill.

Schultz, R., & Beach, S. R. (1999). Caregiving as a risk factor for mortality: The caregiver health effects study. *Journal of the American Medical Association, 282*(23), 2215–2219.

Schunemann, H. J., McCann, S., Grant, B. J., Trevisan, M., Muti, P., & Freudenheim, J. L. (2002). Lung function in relation to intake of carotenoids and other antioxidant vitamins in a population-based study. *American Journal of Epidemiology, 155*(5), 463–471.

Stollman, N., & Raskin, J. (1999). Diagnosis and management of diverticular disease in adults. *The American Journal of Gastroenterology, 94*(11), 3110–3121.

Thomas, D. R., Ashmen, Morley, & Evans (2000). Nutritional management in long term care: Development of a clinical guideline. *Journal of Gerontology, 55A*(12), M725–M734.

Toyonaga, A., Okamatsu, H., Sasaki, K., Kimura, H., Saito, T., Shimizu, S., Fukuizumi, K., Tsuruta, O., Tanikawa, K., & Sata, M. (2000). An epidemiological study on food intake and Helicobacter pylori infection. *Kurume Medical Journal, 47*(1), 25–30.

Watson, Y., Arfken, C., & Birge, S. (1993). Clock completion: An objective screening test for dementia. *Journal of the American Geriatrics Society, 41,* 1235–1240.

Zhang, S., Giovannucci, E., Hunter, D., Rimm, E., Ascherio, A., Colditz, G., Speizer, F., & Willett, W. (2001). Vitamin supplement use and the risk of non-Hodgkin's lymphoma among women and men. *American Journal of Epidemiology, 153*(11), 1056–1063.

–10–

Irritable Bowel Syndrome

Sue E. Meiner

Irritable bowel syndrome (IBS) is a functional disorder of the gastrointestinal system. The definition of "functional" disorder is the presence of symptoms without any organic origin or cause. Functional bowel disorders are variable combinations of chronic or recurrent gastrointestinal (GI) symptoms attributed to all levels of the GI tract that have no structural or biochemical explanation. Without a physiologic indicator, older adults with symptoms of IBS are often misdiagnosed and exposed to treatments that do not relieve the symptoms.

IBS does not discriminate by age or gender, although women seek medical advice more frequently in Western societies than do men, and are diagnosed more frequently. Many older adults are worried that the symptoms of IBS are signs of cancer of the colon. Since it is an illness that crosses all decades of life, the effects on older adults will be examined. This chapter will provide needed information to relieve the anxiety that fear of cancer brings, and thus reduce the symptoms that further exacerbate an episode of IBS in the older adult.

The symptoms of IBS are known to wax and wane in irregular patterns. When psychological stress increases in patients with IBS, the symptoms become exacerbated. Finding that stress increases IBS symptoms, current researchers have delved into identification of a connection between neurochemicals that are found in the brain and the GI tract (Camilleri & Spiller, 2002; Bilhartz & Croft, 2000). The importance of distinguishing IBS from functional diarrhea, constipation, or bloating is necessary because different diagnostic and treatment issues need to be addressed (Thompson, Heaton, Smyth, & Smyth, 2000).

Only a relatively small number of older adults seek medical attention for the symptoms of IBS. Reasons for consulting a health care professional include the number of symptoms, the presence of psychosocial stressors, and the presence of perceived pain. This chapter will explore the symptoms, associations, and current treatments recommended for persons with IBS.

DEFINITIONS

The following narrative definitions are provided to assist in a general understanding of material presented (Porth, 1998). If further assistance is sought, the references at the end of this chapter will provide additional information on IBS.

A *neurotransmitter* is any one of numerous chemicals that modify or result in the transmission of nerve impulses. Neurotransmitters are called catecholamines. These chemicals are the source of bodily activities that require movement, such as dilatation, and constriction. The GI tract's motility requires coordinated activities of neurotransmitters.

Serotonin (5-hydroxytryptamine or 5-HT) is found in the brain and in the GI tract. The serotonin found in the intestinal tissue serves as a neurotransmitter and stimulates the smooth muscles to contract. The role that serotonin plays in the normal physiology of the GI tract suggests that even a minor alteration in serotonergic function might have distressing results for intestinal motility, secretion, and sensation.

Nociceptors are free nerve endings that respond to painful stimuli. They can be stimulated by injury to tissue or by other chemicals in the GI tract that produce an excitatory response.

ETIOLOGY

The exact cause of IBS is unknown. Over the past two decades, several suspected relationships have been inferred. One such relationship involves psychological reasons that have not been proven or eliminated from studies addressing the causes of IBS. Psychologists are unlikely to see IBS patients who are psychologically normal, and thereby draw conclusions that IBS is a psychological disorder. The cognitive and behavioral backgrounds of patients with IBS are currently under study by Drossman (2000) and colleagues. Physiologists are likely to believe the explanation lies in the study of intestinal motility or sensations. Views of health care providers, surgeons, and dietitians offer additional causes or relationships associated with IBS. However a strong link is emerging between the neurochemical serotonin found in the brain and in the GI tract (Thompson, 2002).

In the general population, estimates of the prevalence of symptoms consistent with IBS are approximately 15 percent (Horwitz & Fisher, 2001). The presentation of IBS symptoms accounts for almost 50% of referrals to gastroenterologists. Although 50% of IBS cases are diagnosed before age 35, nearly all are identified by age 50. This makes IBS a chronic condition for older adults. The prevalence among Caucasians outnumbers all other ethnic groups, and women outnumber men 2:1 (Yamada, Alperts, Owyang, Powell, Silverstein, Hasler, et al., 1999).

PATHOPHYSIOLOGY

Gastrointestinal function is controlled by the enteric nervous system, which is contained within the wall of the GI tract, and by the parasympathetic and sympathetic divisions of the autonomic nervous system. The common features of IBS involve altered bowel motility, visceral hypersensitivity with pain, an imbalance in neurotransmitters, possible inflammation or infection (see chapter 6), and a psychosocial element (Porth, 1998). The altered bowel motility can result from physical or psychological stress and ingestion of food. The contractility of the colon is increased in IBS following a high-fat meal.

Visceral hypersensitivity is identified when pain occurs with far less colon bloating than found in non-IBS patients. One explanation was identified by Horwitz and Fisher (2001), as "the sensitivity of receptors in the viscus (sic) is altered through the recruitment of silent nociceptors in response to ischemia, distention, intraluminal contents, infection, or psychiatric factors" (p. 1846). The increased perception of abdominal pain has been identified with distention anywhere in the GI tract and is more frequently associated with the irregular motor activity of the small intestine. This increase in sensitivity to visceral pain doesn't extend to somatic pain. While the perception of pain in the GI tract can be extreme, a high threshold of somatic pain is less likely to be seen in patients with IBS. The processing of the pain stimulus with IBS may take the form of altered patterns of pain referral or increased intensity of visceral pain perception (Bilhartz & Croft, 2000) (Fig. 10.1).

The imbalance in neurotransmitters is thought to be due to increased excitability of the neurons in the dorsal horn of the spinal cord. Catechola-

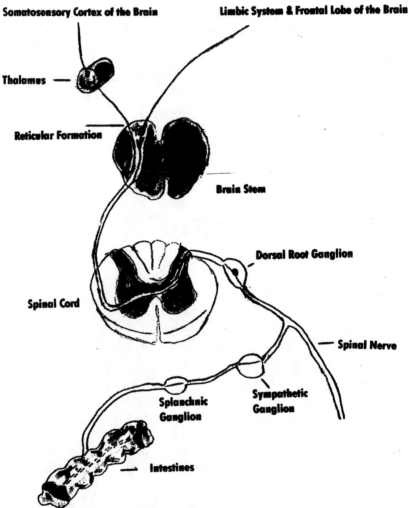

FIGURE 10.1   Neuroanatomic pathway of visceral pain perception.
(Used with permission of Sue E. Meiner)

mines and serotonin are specifically identified with neuronal excitability. This situation suggests a primary central defect of visceral pain processing. Ninety-five percent of the body's serotonin is in the GI tract within the enterochromaffin (EC) cells, neurons, mast cells, and smooth-muscle cells. The function of the EC cells is to reduce salts of chromium or silver to these respective metals. All EC cells are in contact with the GI walls (Gershon, 2002). Serotonin stimulates the extrinsic vagal afferent nerve fibers and the intrinsic enteric afferent nerve fibers. This results in physiological responses such as intestinal secretion and peristaltic reflex. These reflexes can produce symptoms of nausea, vomiting, abdominal pain, and bloating (Gershon, 1999). Although other neurotransmitters are present in gastrointestinal disorders, many current studies have been done on the connection between catecholamines and serotonin on the bowel (Gershon, 2002). This information has led to a treatment option for some older adults with IBS.

Psychosocial. Psychosocial factors include personality, psychological distress, social stress, and to a lesser extent psychiatric disorders which can be identified with the use of self-administered questionnaires. These tools can be helpful in providing the clinician with an indication of the level of the person's distress. Some tools might give false positives due to the physical symptoms of IBS. One of these is the Beck Depression Inventory (Beck, Ward, & Mendelson, 1961), which has items concerning aches and pains, upset stomach, constipation, and changes in appetite. These items are surely going to be scored positively by patients with IBS, thus giving an incorrect evaluation (Creed, 1999; Creed, 2002). This is especially important when depression is suspected in an older adult. If the past medical history of an older adult indicates a diagnosis of IBS or of longstanding symptoms of IBS, the Beck Depression Scale needs to be reviewed with an understanding of the potential false positive finding. Table 10.1 lists commonly used psychosocial instruments that are less likely to be affected by the symptoms of IBS.

When using any of the common psychosocial instruments listed in Table 10.1, attention needs to be given to the higher than normal scores on the STAXI (Speilberger, 1985), and the SCL-90 tests among IBS patients when compared with healthy groups. This is related to the body symptoms categories. The HADS questionnaire provides scores for anxiety and depression separately, while bodily symptoms do not influence the scores (Creed, 2002).

The role of sexual, physical, and emotional abuse and patients with IBS has been speculated for decades. While abuse remains an intensely subjective experience for each individual, it is usually suspected in patients who

TABLE 10.1   Commonly Used Psychosocial Instruments

Dimension to Be Measured	Instrument
Personality	EPI—Eysenck personality inventory
	STAXI—Speilberger trait anxiety inventory
Psychological distress	SCL-90—Hopkins symptom checklist
Illness attitudes and beliefs	IBQ—illness behavior questionnaire
	IAS—illness attitude scale
Psychological distress	GHQ—general health questionnaire
	HADS—hospital anxiety and depression scale

Adapted from: Creed, F. (2002). Relationship between IBS and psychiatric disorders. In M. Camilleri & R. C. Spiller, *Irritable bowel syndrome: Diagnosis and treatment*. Philadelphia: W. B. Saunders.

develop IBS later in life. Self-report questionnaires or structured interviews administered by a clinician are the most frequently used methods of identifying the person who has a history of abuse. Validation of abuse other than self-disclosure is difficult due to the scarcity of reports to family, friends, or police. The association of abuse has been most extensively studied in IBS patients by Drossman, Leserman, and Nachman (1990). The Drossman study found that 50% of the IBS patients had a history of abuse. Talley and colleagues (1994) completed a population-based study that found IBS appearing at a rate three times greater among persons reporting adult or childhood abuse. As patients with a history of abuse and IBS are more likely to have poorer health and may pose a greater challenge in illness management, inquiries about an abusive history should be considered as part of the initial examination. Unfortunately an inquiry about abuse, especially sexual abuse, is most often deferred in the taking of the past medical history of an older adult. Therefore the clinician must be alert and sensitive regarding initiating questions that can elicit appropriate information.

Older adults are frequently faced with multiple losses as their life continues. Often these losses lead to stress that does not abate before the next loss. Then the stress level increases twofold. Each new stress creates additional levels of stress and then stress-related illnesses such as IBS occur or reoccur with each new stressful situation. An example is the recent widow who loses the family pet, then needs to move out of the family home into an apartment due to an inability to maintain a house. She has lost a husband, pet, home, and many possessions that cannot go into an apartment. Relocation stress is added to all of the other stresses.

Physical. Criteria for identification of IBS is based upon complaints of at least three months of continuous or recurrent symptoms of abdominal pain or discomfort that is relieved by defecation or is associated with a change in frequency or consistency of stool. A minimum of two other symptoms, in combination with disturbed defecation, commonly persist for at least 25% of the time. These characteristics can include altered stool frequency, altered stool form (e.g., lumpy or hard, or loose or watery), altered stool passage (e.g., straining, urgency, or feeling of incomplete evacuation), passage of mucus, with bloating or a feeling of abdominal distention (Hasler & Owyang, 1999; Hahn, Watson, Yan, Gunput, & Heuijerjans, 1998). See the following three tables for criteria used to diagnose IBS as presented by different diagnosticians. See Table 10.2, the Manning criteria, Table 10.3, the Kruis criteria, and Table 10.4, the ROME criteria.

Treatment classifications. Adult and older adult patients should be classified as having mild, moderate, or severe IBS. The classifications differ by the severity of physiologic symptoms, psychosocial associations, illness behavior, and activity disruption symptoms. Mild IBS is the predominant

TABLE 10.2   The Manning Criteria for the Diagnosis of Irritable Bowel Syndrome

Looser stools at onset of pain

More frequent stools at onset of pain

Abdominal distention

Passage of mucus per rectum

Sense of incomplete evacuation

From: Manning, A. P., Thompson, W. G., Heaton, K. W., et al. (1978). Towards positive diagnosis of the irritable bowel. *British Medical Journal, 2,* 653.

TABLE 10.3   The Kruis Criteria for the Diagnosis of Irritable Bowel Syndrome

Abdominal pain plus flatulence plus irregularity

Symptoms duration > 2 years

Diarrhea and constipation

From: Kruis, W., Thieme, C. H., Weinzierl, M., et al. (1984). A diagnostic score for irritable bowel syndrome: Its value in exclusion of organic disease. *Gastroenterology, 87,* 1.

TABLE   10.4   ROME Diagnostic Criteria for Irritable Bowel Syndrome

Continuous or recurrent symptoms for at least three months of both of the following:

1. Abdominal pain or discomfort that is relieved with defecation and/or associated with a change in frequency of stool and/or associated with a change in consistency of stool
2. Three or more of the following, at least one fourth of occasions or days:
   Altered stool frequency (more than three bowel movements per day or fewer than three bowel movements per week)
   Altered stool form
   Altered stool passage
   Passage of mucus
   Bloating or feeling of abdominal distention

From: Thompson, W. G., Creed, F., Drossman, D. A., et al. (1992). Functional bowel disease and functional abdominal pain. *Gastroenterology International*, 5:75.

form of this functional bowel disease. Patients with mild disease have infrequent symptoms that do not result in significant psychological or functional impairment. These patients can be treated with education, reassurance, and a few dietary changes. Patients with moderate symptoms have intermittent functional impairments and more psychological distress from their symptoms. They are frequently able to relate symptoms to psychological stressors or to specific dietary indiscretions. These patients may require directed pharmacotherapy, behavioral therapy, and psychotherapy in addition to the treatments described for patients with mild disease. Patients with severe disease have frequent disruption of daily activities and can't relate symptoms to specific physiologic changes such as diet or activity. Often these patients have associated psychological disturbances and find fault with the primary care provider and the treatment options offered, especially when psychological referrals are made (Bilhartz & Croft, 2000). Many older adults may not want to change their current lifestyle even with symptoms that are so troubling that medical care is sought. A careful explanation of the potential improvement in their quality of life should be made when a suggested dietary regimen is rejected by the older adult.

GENERAL NURSING CARE

IBS is a common problem facing primary care providers and nurses working with patients in a primary care setting. Primary care of persons with IBS ranges from the initial contact, comprehensive assessment, continuity and coordination of care, and patient-centered focus. Initial presentations are of an undifferentiated illness, with diffuse symptoms that may be in evolution at the time of the visit. The symptoms can range from physical signs, psychological issues, and social problems. Personal continuity and coordination are essential with care of the IBS patient. This entails placing the patient with a provider of care that will be able to continue to see this patient over time. With so many health care systems using referral networks, the primary care provider and nursing staff need to maintain coordinated services between secondary care, referrals, and social services as needed. If the person is over age 65 and is using Medicare, provider selection could be a problem. Some Medicare recipients have elected to have medical care provided through an HMO network for senior care. Attention is needed in selecting an appropriate provider within a network of approved providers. Patient-centered care includes health promotion, illness prevention, and education aimed at the interplays between the physical, psychological, and social problems associated with IBS.

Assessment. In addition to a carefully and sympathetically taken history, the physical examination is important in seeking other signs which might have implications for the seriousness of the underlying condition. Anemia, obvious weight loss, an abdominal mass, rectal bleeding, and/or increased tenderness or abnormal findings on rectal examination need further evaluation. These cardinal symptoms of organic bowel disease need to be differentiated from IBS symptoms. Diagnostic tests include a complete blood count (CBC) and an erythrocyte sedimentation rate (ESR) to rule out anemia and inflammation. When diarrhea is present, a stool culture and analysis for occult blood, ova and parasites, and bacteria are recommended. Older adults with new symptoms should have a sigmoidoscopy with air insufflation and a barium enema with contrast to exclude other GI tract disorders. When persistent constipation is the problem, evaluate for hypothyroidism. A three-week trial of lactose-free meals can rule out lactose intolerance as a cause of some symptoms.

Planning. After organic bowel disease is eliminated from the diagnosis, planning of continued care is appropriate. With continuity of care as a goal, the patient with IBS symptoms may need to be seen at several follow-up visits over a few weeks and months to determine the true nature of the GI illness. Over time the symptoms will provide a pattern that fits the definition of IBS, and then patient specific treatment can be instituted.

NURSING DIAGNOSES AND PLAN OF CARE

1. Bowel incontinence related to dietary habits, chronic diarrhea, intestinal pressure, or rapid transit of feces

Definition: change in normal bowel habits characterized by involuntary passage of stool

Plan of Care: determine current pattern of elimination and promote control or management of the underlying cause (Doenges, Moorhouse, & Geissler-Murr, 2000).

2. Diarrhea related to high stress levels and anxiety; GI illness symptom

   Definition: passage of loose unformed stools

   Plan of Care: Communicate with the patient until verbalization of understanding of the causative factors and rationale for treatment regimen including reduction of stress (Doenges, Moorhouse, & Geissler-Murr, 2000).

3. Constipation related to irregular defecation habits; insufficient physical activity; GI illness symptom

   Definition: decrease in normal frequency of defecation accompanied by difficult or incomplete passage of stool and/or passage of excessively hard, dry stool

   Plan of Care: Assist the patient to establish/regain normal pattern of bowel functioning using appropriate IBS protocols and continue to monitor over time (Doenges, Moorhouse, & Geissler-Murr, 2000).

4. Pain, chronic related to chronic physical/psychological disability

   Definition: unpleasant sensory and emotional experience arising from actual or potential tissue stimulus

   Plan of Care: assess etiology/precipitating factors; evaluate emotional/physical components of individual situation; determine cultural factors involved; assess with an understanding of methods to heal by developing a sense of internal control by being responsible for own treatment, and by obtaining the information and tools to accomplish this task (Doenges, Moorhouse, & Geissler-Murr, 2000).

5. Coping, ineffective, related to inadequate level of confidence in ability to cope/perception of control

   Definition: inability to form a valid appraisal of the stressors, inadequate choices of practiced responses, and/or inability to use available resources.

   Plan of Care: assess current functional capacity and note how it is affecting the individual's coping ability; assess level of anxiety and coping on an ongoing basis (Doenges, Moorhouse, & Geissler-Murr, 2000).

6. Self-esteem, chronic low, related to negative perceptions of how others view him or her

Definition: longstanding negative self-evaluation/feelings about self or self-capabilities

Plan of Care: refer or conduct a treatment program to promote changes in self-evaluation; demonstrate behaviors/lifestyle changes to promote positive self-esteem (Doenges, Moorhouse, & Geissler-Murr, 2000).

INTERVENTIONS, TREATMENTS, ALTERNATIVE TREATMENTS

Interventions. The use of reassurance therapy should not begin until all data are examined and a diagnosis of IBS is made. Explaining the pathophysiology of the symptoms is a prerequisite for effective reassurance therapy. Although the pathophysiology is poorly understood, current thinking in regard to motility abnormalities and visceral hypersensitivity in the intestinal tract should be described. Reassurance will only be successful if the patient perceives that the health care providers understand the basis of the symptoms, a sense of urgency to eliminate the symptoms is not alarming, and empathy toward the plight of the patient is felt (Jones, 2002).

Treatment. A diary of food intake and symptoms can be useful in identifying foods that may be associated with IBS. Patients often report an exacerbation of symptoms after the consumption of certain foods. Some patients benefit from avoiding or limiting their intake of caffeine, alcohol, fatty foods, gas-producing vegetables, or products containing sorbitol (e.g., sugarless candies and gum). Constipating foods should be avoided when constipation is the main feature of IBS. Adding 20 to 30 grams of fiber every day may help with constipation and occasionally improve the symptom of diarrhea.

When suspected food intolerance exacerbates symptoms, an exclusionary diet can be offered. This diet requires full commitment by the patient and may take several weeks to complete. It begins with a seven-day diet consisting of one meat, one fruit, rice and water. If symptoms of IBS remain, food intolerance is not considered a serious element of the patient's symptoms and the diet may be discontinued. However, if the symptoms were reduced or eliminated, then the exclusionary diet should be continued. Foods may be introduced one at a time each day. Any foods added that provoke symptoms of IBS are then excluded. This plan could produce a diet that eliminates symptoms. See Table 10.5, for a list of foods that are on the exclusionary diet protocol (Atkinson & Hunter, 2002; Parker et al., 1995).

TABLE 10.5   List of Foods Suspected of Stimulating IBS Symptoms and to Be Avoided as Part of an Exclusionary Diet

Grains:	Vegetables:	Fruits:
Wheat	Onions	Citrus
Rye	Cabbage	Rhubarb
Barley	Sprouts	Apples
Oats	Potatoes	Bananas
Corn	Peas	
Rice		
Meats:	Dairy:	Other:
Beef	Milk	Coffee
Pork	Cheese	Tea
Chicken	Eggs	Nuts
	Butter	Chocolate
		Preservatives
		Yeast

Adapted from Parker, T. J., Naylor, S. J., Riordan, A. M., et al. (1995). Management of patients with food intolerance in irritable bowel syndrome: The development and use of an exclusion diet. *Journal of Human Nutrition and Diet, 8,* 159–166.

Counseling. Counseling may be useful with IBS patients, particularly when there is a substantial interplay between social, psychological, and physical factors. Formal psychotherapy may be beneficial for some patients, while not for others.

Cognitive therapy. Cognitive therapies modify the patient's maladaptive beliefs about their pain by replacing that belief with a more realistic view of their health state. This type of therapy focuses upon improving the patient's awareness of the association between the stressors and the pain experienced. Keeping a diary to reflect back on events and symptoms can lead to identification of the causes and then a modification of the stimulating behavior to prevent a recurrence (Greene & Blanchard, 1994).

Behavioral therapy. Behavioral treatments focus upon changing the patient's behavior in relation to the pain experienced by IBS. An example of the need for this type of intervention is the patient who avoids social events because of the fear that restrooms will be too far away from the event area. Fearing an uncontrollable bowel movement, these patients often stay home (Lynch & Zamble, 1989).

Combination therapy. The use of cognitive and behavioral therapy together is recognized as superior to the limited benefits of behavioral therapy alone, and has demonstrated greater effectiveness than cognitive therapy alone. One behavioral therapy that is used with cognitive therapy is biofeed-back. This is especially beneficial with patients suffering from idiopathic constipation (Toner, 1998; Blanchard, Greene, & Scharff, 1993).

Abuse counseling. The use of interpersonal therapies in abuse counseling is helpful in some instances where the patient is willing to examine the relationship between the symptoms of IBS and marital distress, family friction, or a previous history of abuse or unresolved bereavements. These unresolved issues can lead to the cycle of pain, distress, and disability with IBS. Once the identification of the stressor is made, an understanding of the effect the stressors have on the patient's health and quality of life can be made. Support for making the necessary changes to improve the thought patterns, and work toward emotional healing are the goals of interpersonal therapy (Drossman, Talley, Leserman, Olden, & Barreiro, 1995; Guthrie, Moorey, & Margison, 1999).

Elder abuse should be suspected and action taken to prevent it from continuing when an older adult is seen in a medical office with signs and symptoms of IBS and physical signs of neglect or mistreatment. Counseling is essential when the older adult verbalizes an acceptable reason for the suspected abuse. Abuse by family members is often not reported by an older adult.

Pharmacotherapy. Drug therapy should be aimed at the predominant symptom of IBS, and should be monitored regularly to determine its success. Adjustments are often needed if symptoms change or become exacerbated. If you are a staff nurse, notify the primary care provider of the change, and provide any new patient teaching as indicated. If you are a nurse practitioner, assess for needed modification in pharmacotherapy plan, and proceed accordingly.

Diarrhea-predominant IBS responds well to a loperamide 4 mg tablet or capsule for a loose stool, followed by 2 mg after subsequent loose stools, not to exceed a daily dosage of 8 mg (self directed) or 16 mg by prescription. Over-the-counter liquid loperamide comes as 1 mg in 5 ml, with the same daily dosage limits. Prescription medication for control of diarrhea is a time-limited treatment. Diphenoxylate HCl and atropine sulfate (Lomotil), 1 to 2 tablets four times a day until the diarrhea stops, not to exceed 8 tablets in 24 hours, is the normal dosage. Since this medication can become habituating, a limit to its continuous use must be evaluated by the primary care provider (Hoole, Pickard, Ouimette, Lohr, & Powell, 1999).

Constipation-predominant IBS responds well to dietary changes that include adding bulking agents to the daily diet. While bran can be used to increase the intake of dietary fiber, calcium polycabophil, psyllium, and methylcellulose result in less bloating than bran. Osmotic laxatives may be helpful. Magnesium preparations are more beneficial than aluminum preparations. Aluminum preparations often result in more constipation than less. Other laxatives with polyethylene glycol (PEG) may be helpful.

Distention, bloating, or pain-predominant IBS responds to antispasmodics and GI TRACT smooth-muscle relaxants. However, antispasmodics are not recommended for treatment of IBS in older adults because of the anticholinergic side effects of these medications (Kennedy-Malone, Fletcher, & Plank, 2000). Low-dose tricyclic antidepressants have been found to be effective as well. When these symptoms are combined with diarrhea or constipation, advice is needed on a one-on-one basis with a primary care provider.

Intestinal gas (flatus) is extremely common and distressful for most sufferers of IBS. This is often accompanied by audible bowel sounds (borborygmi). While non-IBS individuals pass flatus several times a day, it is usually controlled and done during bowel movements or bathroom stops. The IBS patient often has little control over timing of the release of flatus even though the frequency of flatus does not differ with that of non-IBS individuals. This adds to the perceived embarrassment of borborygmi and frequent trips to the bathroom when diarrhea is the predominant symptom. One rationale for the impaired release of flatus is thought to be a hypersensitivity to physiological volumes of intestinal gas. Exclusionary diets have been found to reduce the loss of control of flatus by reducing the amount of fermentation by the colonic flora and thus reduction in the release of flatus (Furne & Levitt, 1996; Levitt, Furne, & Olsson, 1996; Whorwell, P.J., 2000). See Table 10.5, for a list of foods on the exclusionary diet.

The use of selective serotonin reuptake inhibitors (SSRIs) is becoming a treatment of choice with constipation and pain predominant IBS. The relationship of serotonin and the GI tract has led new research in the direction of using individual agents in the SSRI category such as buspirone, paroxetine, and citalopram for treatment of IBS in specific patients. These drugs have been used in depression treatment with a high degree of success. The uses of SSRIs in disorders of the GI tract are finding success with smaller doses than those used in depression treatment. However, these drugs must be used on a continuous rather than an as-needed basis, so they are reserved for those IBS patients with frequent recurring or continual symptoms (Apter & Allen, 1999; Clouse, 1994; Kim & Camilleri, 2000).

Probiotics are microorganisms which exert health benefits greater than the basic nutritional source alone. Lactobacillus plantarum is a probiotic that is thought to replace a deficiency of normal colon bacteria. When taken in sufficient quantity, this probiotic has been shown to reduce flatus and bloating better than placebo. Patients were noted to have an improved overall GI function after 12 months of probiotic therapy (Noback, Johansson, Molin, et al., 2000).

Pain management may provide another source of therapy. Chronic pain syndromes can be associated with IBS and require evaluation and treatment according to the severity of the symptoms.

Alternative Treatments. Hypnosis has been shown to be particularly effective in IBS patients, although it is labor-intensive and can be expensive. Identifying an appropriate hypnotherapist might pose difficulties in some communities (Whorwell, Prior, & Colgan, 1987). Other complementary therapies such as Chinese medicines have been shown in carefully-designed studies to have significant benefit in IBS patients.

Bodywork and exercise are important therapies for persons with IBS. Relaxation therapy in groups or self-directed is beneficial in reduction of stress by releasing muscle tension. Relaxation is especially useful when anxiety, fatigue, and sleep disturbances are present. Breathing exercises can help release tension. Often people breathe in an erratic and shallow manner using only the upper part of the chest. When deeper and more regular breathing can be achieved, an improved mood results and falling asleep can be easier. Unless contraindicated, moderate continuous exercise of walking for 20 to 30 minutes at least three days a week is the minimum amount of physical activity recommended for healthy gastric motility. Alternative exercise programs include riding a stationary bike, doing abdominal and pelvic floor muscle strengthening exercises, and range-of-motion (passive and active) exercises, which can be beneficial to those who are less mobile. When more activities can be undertaken, the benefits of exercise will become apparent in decreased episodes of fecal incontinence, more normal bowel movements, and a reduction in the need for laxatives (Adelman & Daly, 2001).

HEALTH PROMOTION AND QUALITY OF LIFE ISSUES

Health promotion includes normal activities and instrumental activities of daily living. Illness prevention is associated with health promotion. Therefore, preventing repeated episodes of IBS is important to those concepts. Socialization is a significant part of life for most people, and is especially important for older adults with large blocks of time to fill. A strong subjective component is associated with quality of life statements.

Health related quality of life is often defined according to physical functioning, emotional well-being, and general health perceptions. The separation of general quality of life and health related quality of life is difficult. Due to the subjective nature of this concept, an instrument to examine the perception of quality of life was developed by Ferrans (1996). This objective assessment is connected to a person's judgments, values, life experiences, and satisfaction with aspects of life. The four quality of life domains examined are 1) health and functioning, 2) psychospiritual, 3) socioeconomic, and 4) family (Hahn, Yan, & Strassels, 1999). Nurses can use the information gained from an objective assessment of quality of life measures to plan, implement, and evaluate interventions for older adults with IBS. Identifying ways to reduce the stress of daily living and control the symptoms of IBS can go a long way in achieving a higher quality of life (Lubkin & Larsen, 2002).

HOME MANAGEMENT AND SELF-CARE ISSUES

Stress reduction techniques need to be practiced at home especially when emotional situations are present. Recommend that food products known to irritate the bowel not be purchased or stored in the residence to prevent eating foods that stimulate symptoms. Label reading before buying food is essential when screening foods for bowel irritating ingredients. Even inactive ingredients in over-the-counter medicines may cause bowel irritation. When bulking agents are used, sufficient water must be taken with the agent. Using the powder forms of bulking agents with large quantities of water or juice is preferred over tablets that may be taken with only a small amount of water. Constipation can become much worse if insufficient water is consumed with the bulking agents. The dehydration factor for older adults is always a concern that needs attention. Drinking six to eight glasses (8 ounces) of water a day is vital to well-being.

FOLLOW-UP CARE

With chronic IBS patients, a positive relationship between primary care provider and clinician is mutually beneficial. Dietary intervention and stress-reduction techniques should be reviewed and evaluated. In patients with newly diagnosed IBS, evaluation of persistent symptoms is needed because IBS is a diagnosis of exclusion.

Follow-up screening at three- and six-week intervals is important when symptoms continue or new ones appear. If diarrhea persists, an assessment of the quantity and quality of the diarrhea is needed. A timed stool collection for volume, osmolarity, electrolytes, laxatives, and fecal fat can be done. Stool volumes of more than 400 cc per day suggest malabsorption or secretory diarrhea. If constipation persists, a colonic transit testing can be done.

CONCLUSION

Problems with the digestive system, especially IBS, cause personal, family, social, and business concerns for the sufferer. Family outings are cancelled, social invitations are refused, and sports activities, trips, and business events are interrupted frequently when a flare-up of IBS occurs. This functional GI disorder is complex and requires in-depth information from the patient in order to help reduce or relieve the symptoms. It may require a nutritional and/or counseling referral. Some prescribed medications are available to help with specific symptoms but not all exacerbations respond. Some over-the-counter drugs can be recommended according to the classification and predominant features presented by each individual IBS patient. Caution must be exercised in ruling out nonfunctional or organic causes of the intestinal symptoms before the diagnosis of IBS is made. Nonfunctional or organic causes need evaluation immediately due to the potentially rapid advance of some diseases of the colon. Once the diagnosis of IBS is made, the treatments described in this chapter can be considered. The following resources may be helpful for patients and caregivers:

International Foundation for Functional Gastrointestinal Disorders
P.O. Box 17864; Milwaukee, WI 53217; (888) 964-2001
iffgd@iffgd.org www.iffgd.org

National Digestive Diseases Information Clearinghouse
Irritable Bowel Syndrome
2 Information Way; Bethesda, MD 20892-3570
ndic@info.niddk.nih.gov
www.niddk.nih.gov/health/digest/pubs/irrbowel/irrbowel.htm

REFERENCES

Adelman, A. M., & Daly, M. P. (2001). *20 common problems in geriatrics*. New York: McGraw-Hill Publishing.

Care of the Older Adult With Gastrointestinal Problems

174Care of the Older Adult With Gastrointestinal Problems

Hahn, B., Yan, S., & Strassels, S. (1999). Impact of irritable bowel syndrome on quality of life and resource use in the United States and United Kingdom. *Digestion*, 60(1), 77–81.

Hasler, W. L., & Owyang, C. (1999). Irritable bowel syndrome. In T. Yamada et al. (Eds.), *Textbook of gastroenterology*, Vol. 2, 3rd ed. Philadelphia: Lippincott Williams & Wilkins.

Hoole, A. J., Pickard, C. G., Ouimette, R., Lohr, J. A., & Powell, W. I. (1999). *Patient care guidelines for nurse practitioners*, 5th ed. Philadelphia: Lippincott.

Horwitz, B. J., & Fisher, R. S. (2001). The irritable bowel syndrome. *The New England Journal of Medicine*, 344(24), 1846–1850.

Jones, R. (2002). Managing IBS: The perspective from primary care. In M. Camilleri & R. C. Spiller, *Irritable bowel syndrome: Diagnosis and treatment*. Philadelphia: W. B. Saunders.

Kennedy-Malone, L., Fletcher, K. R., & Plank, L. M. (2000). *Management guidelines for gerontological nurse practitioners*. Philadelphia: F. A. Davis.

Kim, D. Y., & Camilleri, M. (2000). Serotonin: A modulator of the brain-gut connection. *American Journal of Gastroenterology*, 95, 2698–2709.

Kruis, W., Thieme, C. H., Weinzierl, M., et al. (1984). A diagnostic score for irritable bowel syndrome: Its value in exclusion of organic disease. *Gastroenterology*, 87, 1.

Levitt, M. D., Furne, J., & Olsson, S. (1996). The relation of passage of gas and abdominal bloating to colonic gas production. *Annals of Internal Medicine*, 124, 422–424.

Lubkin, I. M., & Larsen, P. D. (2002). *Chronic illness: Impact and interventions*, 5th ed. Boston: Jones and Bartlett Publishers.

Lynch, P. M., & Zamble, E. A. (1989). Controlled behavioral treatment for irritable bowel syndrome. *Behavioral Therapies*, 20, 509–523.

Manning, A. P., Thompson, W. G., Heaton, K. W., et al. (1978). Towards positive diagnosis of the irritable bowel. *British Medical Journal*, 2, 653.

Noback, S., Johansson, M. L., Molin, G., et al. Alteration of intestinal microflora is associated with reduction in abdominal blasting and pain in patients with irritable bowel syndrome. *American Journal of Gastroenterology*, 95, 1231–1238.

Parker, T. J., Naylor, S. J., Riordan, A. M., et al. (1995). Management of patients with food intolerance in irritable bowel syndrome: The development and use of an exclusion diet. *Journal of Human Nutrition and Diet*, 8, 159–166.

Porth, C. M. (1998). *Pathophysiology: Concepts of altered health states*, 5th ed. Philadelphia: Lippincott.

Speilberger, C. D. (1983). *Manual for the State-Trait Anxiety Inventory (Form Y)*. Palo Alto, CA: Consulting Psychologists Press.

Talley, N. J., Fett, S. L., Zinsmeister, A. R., et al. (1994). Gastrointestinal tract symptoms and self-reported abuse: A population-based study. *Gastroenterology*, 107, 1040–1049.

Thompson, W. G. (2002). A world-view of IBS. In M. Camilleri & R. C. Spiller, *Irritable bowel syndrome: Diagnosis and treatment*. Philadelphia: W. B. Saunders.

Thompson, W. G., Creed, F., Drossman, D. A., et al. (1992). Functional bowel disease and functional abdominal pain. *Gastroenterology International*, 5, 75.

Thompson, W. G., Heaton, K. W., Smyth, T., & Smyth, C. (2000). Irritable bowel syndrome in general practice: Prevalence, management and referral. *Gut, 46,* 78–82.
Toner, B. B. (1998). Cognitive behavioral group therapy for patients with irritable bowel syndrome. *International Journal of Group Psychotherapy, 48,* 215–243.
Whorwell, P. J. (2000). The problem of gas in the irritable bowel syndrome. *American Journal of Gastroenterology, 95,* 1618–1619.
Whorwell, P. J., Prior, A., & Colgan, S. M. (1987). Hypnotherapy in severe irritable bowel syndrome: Further experience. *Gut, 4,* 423–425.
Yamada, T., Alperts, D. H., Owyang, C., Powell, D. W., Silverstein, F. E., Hasler, W. L., Traber, P. G., & Tierney, W. M. (1999). *Handbook of gastroenterology.* Philadelphia: Lippincott Williams & Wilkins.

–11–

Diverticular Disease

D. Sue Clarren

Diverticular disease is of importance in the older adult, presenting in clients over 40 years of age and significantly increasing in incidence and severity with age. The average age at onset of diverticulitis is between 60 to 70 years. It is the most common disease of the colon in the United States (Oeffinger, 2000). This disease presents with many different signs and symptoms that require many diagnostic and aggressive therapies with significant morbidity in the older adult (Deckman & Cheskin, 1993). Diverticulosis is the presence of pouches of mucosa and submucosa in the large intestine. These pouches occur between the circular muscles of the colon. Uncomplicated diverticulitis is noted when an inflammation and subsequent peridiverticular infection of one or more of the pouches occurs (Bilhartz & Croft, 2000). Definitions of terms related to diverticular disease can be found in Table 11.1.

ETIOLOGY

Diverticular disease is common in western societies with the highest incidence in the United States, Europe, and Australia. It is uncommon for diverticular disease to affect persons under 40 years of age (Dunphy & Winland-Brown, 2001). It affects approximately 5–10% of the population over 45 years of age, with the incidence and severity increasing with age and approaches 80% of persons over the age of 85 (Mirsha, 2002). It is

178 Care of the Older Adult With Gastrointestinal Problems

TABLE 11.1   Definitions Related to Diverticular Disease

The following definitions taken from Digestive Health and Disease: A Glossary, from the National Digestive Diseases Information Clearinghouse in 1986 are provided to assist the reader.

Abscess: A localized pocket of pus.
Anastomosis: The surgical formation of a passageway between any two spaces or hollow organs in the body.
Bloating: A feeling of fullness in the abdomen, often occurring after a meal.
Colonoscopy: A long, flexible, narrow endoscope passed through the anus to look into the colon.
Colostomy: The surgical procedure connecting an opening in the colon to a surgically created hole on the body's surface.**Computerized tomography (CT) scanning:** A diagnostic procedure in which the X-ray source rotates around the patient so that an X-ray beam is sent through the patient from many different angles. The X-rays are read by a computer, which constructs three-dimensional images of the body. CT is a painless procedure.
Constipation: Infrequent and/or difficult passage of stools.
Diarrhea: A condition in which bowel movements are passed more often than usual and in a more or less liquid state.
Dietary Fiber: The indigestible, nonstarch material, such as hemicellulose, plant gums, pectins, celluloses found in the cell walls of plants. Dietary fiber is found in a wide variety of plant foods, including whole grain breads and cereals, fresh fruits and vegetables, and nuts. Because dietary fiber resists digestion in the gastrointestinal tract, it accounts for a significant portion of the solid matter in bowel movements.
Distention: A visible increase in the waistline, often occurring after meals.
Diverticula: Plural of diverticulum.
Diverticulitis: A condition in which diverticula become inflamed.
Diverticulosis: A condition in which small sacs (diverticula) form in the wall of the colon. This condition is common among older people.
Diverticulum: A small sac that forms on the wall of a hollow organ (usually the colon).
Enterostomal therapy (ET) nurse: A nurse skilled in caring for and teaching ostomy patients.
Feces: Solid body wastes, passed as bowel movements.
Fiber: The part of a plant that is not digested. Fiber plays a role in controlling the consistency of stool and the speed at which it is moved through the digestive system.
Fistula: An abnormal hollow connection between two internal organs or between an internal organ and the outside of the body.
Flatus: Gas that is passed by the rectum.
Inflammation: A condition in which the body is trying to respond to localized injury or destruction of tissues. All or some of these signs are present: redness, heat, swelling, pain, and loss of function.
Ostomy: A surgical procedure in which a new body opening is created. Usually refers to an opening in the abdomen for the discharge of stool or urine.

TABLE 11.1 *(continued)*

Peristalsis: Progressive wavelike muscular contractions that move materials through the upper GI tract.
Peritonitis: Inflammation of the lining of the abdominal cavity (peritoneum), usually due to intestinal perforation.
Stoma: An artificial opening, for example, an opening in the abdominal wall created by surgery.
Stool: Feces; the waste matter discharged from the anus.

---

estimated that only 20% of patients with diverticula will develop symptomatic diverticulitis (Mirsha, 2002).

In earlier times more men developed diverticular disease than women, although recent studies indicate a similar incidence in men and women (Ferzoco, Raptopoulos, & Silen, 1998). In the United States 90–95% of adults with diverticulosis have involvement of the sigmoid colon (Fig. 11.1), in contrast to Asian countries where 70% have involvement of the right colon. The reason for this is not known (Oeffinger, 2000).

There is no known cause for diverticular disease. It is thought that the change in the dietary habits of the 20th century to a diet low in residue and fiber to be a major contributing cause for the increase in diverticular disease. In the United States from 1909 to 1975, crude fiber intake fell by 28% (Deckman & Cheskin, 1993). Vegetarians who consume more dietary fiber than nonvegetarians have a lower incidence of diverticular disease (Deckman & Cheskin, 1993). A diet high in fiber produces a bulky stool mass that requires a shorter time to pass through the colon. The colon absorbs water from the stool mass for a shorter time maintaining most of the bulk and moisture of the stool. Therefore the stool mass is propelled forward with less resistance. The bulk of the stool mass enlarges the diameter of the colon. The less resistance in propulsion and the larger colon diameter means less colonic segmentation is needed to push the bulky stool through. Thus, intraluminal pressures are not increased. Just the opposite happens when less fiber is ingested. The stool mass is small and does not distend the bowel, and transit time passing through the intestine is increased, causing the stool mass to become hard and dry. More intraluminal pressure is needed to push the stool through the intestines. Older adults frequently drink less water than is recommended each day due to a decline in their thirst mechanism. This decrease in thirst and the subsequent diminished intake of fluids leads to less moisture in the stool as it progresses through the intestines. When less fluid and less bulk

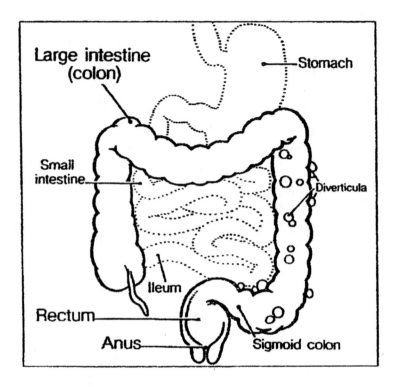

FIGURE 11.1   Large intestine with diverticula.
National Digestive Diseases Information Clearinghouse (1991).

or fiber is ingested routinely, the stool takes on a very hard and dry characteristic. This creates constipation that can evolve into a stool impaction if not treated appropriately. If the older person fails to report this to the nurse or health care provider, an impaction can lead to an emergency situation.

There are several other contributing factors. Suppressing the urge to defecate causes the stool mass transit time to increase, giving the bowel more time to absorb the water, drying out the stool mass and requiring greater segmentation and increased intracolonic pressure to evacuate the stool. Decreased activity/mobility decreases the muscle tone of the abdomen, decreasing transit time and increasing intraluminal pressure. Inadequate daily fluid intake also dries the stool mass requiring more pressure to move the stool mass through the colon. In the elderly an increasing weakness of the bowel muscle caused by aging also slows peristalsis and the transit time of a stool mass.

PATHOLOGY

Diverticulosis is the condition of having diverticula in the colon. Diverticula are a result of increased intracolic pressure causing herniation of colonic mucosa. A diverticulum shows preference for a point of relative weakness in the muscularis, usually where the branches of the marginal artery penetrate the colonic wall. The diverticula are thin mucosal structure sacs with narrow necks. The sigmoid colon is the most common site because it is narrow and the intraluminal pressure is usually greater (Bilhartz & Croft, 2000).

Diverticulosis is usually asymptomatic. Many people do not even know they have diverticulosis. Frequently it is discovered secondarily by radiological studies of the colon for other reasons. If symptoms are present, they are intermittent. Lower left quadrant (LLQ) pain that sometimes becomes worse after eating and relieved after a bowel movement or flatus, and alterations in elimination patterns such as constipation or constipation alternating with diarrhea and abdominal distention are commom. Clients with diverticulosis sometimes present with painless, sudden, and copious rectal bleeding. This bleeding may be the result of a blood vessel eroding at a diverticulum area (Bilhartz & Croft, 2000).

Diverticulitis is the condition in which a diverticulum becomes inflamed. This inflammation is often caused by the retention of undigested food and bacteria (fecalith) in the diverticulum. This mass can disrupt the blood flow. Fecaliths may be related to slow transit times in the affected bowel related to decreased bulk and increased localized intraluminal pressure, especially after meals. A diverticulum has lost its muscular layer and cannot expel the fecalith. This leads to distention of the diverticulum and possible diverticular sac perforation, producing pericolonic inflammation and abscess formation. The abscess usually walls itself off. If an abscess ruptures into the peritoneal cavity, peritonitis usually does not occur because the obstructing material (fecalith) prevents fecal material from entering the peritoneal cavity by sealing off the neck of the diverticulum (Fig. 11.2). However, when a uninflammed diverticulum ruptures it allows leakage of bowel contents into the peritoneal cavity because the neck of the diverticulum is not obstructed. This is called free colonic perforation and causes the serious complication of peritonitis (Bilhartz & Croft, 2000).

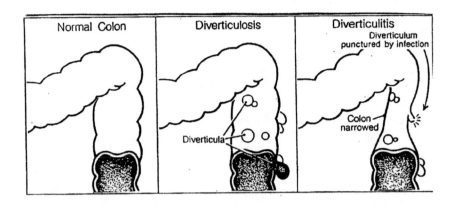

FIGURE 11.2   Diverticulosis in the colon.
National Digestive Diseases Information Clearinghouse (1991).

Classic signs and symptoms of diverticulitis are LLQ pain, fever, and leukocytosis. The onset of pain is usually abrupt, intermittent, without radiation, and unrelated to eating or activity. Nausea and vomiting are also frequently reported.

On physical examination, tenderness and rebound tenderness with guarding can be palpated in the LLQ. Sometimes a firm fixed mass can also be palpated. This is usually an abscess. Bowel sounds may be normal, hypoactive, hyperactive, or absent. Other symptoms may be present involving other organs if a fistula has developed (Table 11.2). The fistula may allow colon air and feces to pass through to the affected organ. A colovesical fistula (an opening between the colon and urinary bladder) may present

TABLE 11.2   Frequency of Symptoms in Diverticulitis

Sign or Symptom	Frequency in Presentation (%)
Pain in Left Lower Quadrant	93–100
Fever	57–100
Leukocytosis	58–83
Nausea	20
Fixed Tenderness (LLQ)	20
Urinary symptoms	10

Bilhartz & Croft (2000) and Oeffinger (2000).

with pneumaturia (passing air with urine) or fecaluria (fecal material in urine), colovaginal fistula (opening between colon and vagina) may present with a vaginal discharge of feces and gas, or a colocutaneous fistula (opening between colon and subcutaneous tissue) may present with subcutaneous emphysema and soft tissue infection.

The elderly and/or immunocompromised patient should be suspect for acute diverticulitis if the patient presents with new onset of LLQ pain, low-grade fever, local tenderness, and elevated white blood cell count (WBC). However it is important to note that these two groups of patients may often present without the usual signs and symptoms. The pain may not be localized, and fever and elevated WBC may be absent. This makes making the diagnosis difficult, but for these high-risk groups it is crucial to diagnose quickly so that effective treatment may be started.

After taking a thorough history and completing a physical exam, the physician may make the diagnosis of mild diverticulitis. If the patient is presenting with systemic signs and symptoms then further evaluation is done with the following laboratory tests and radiological studies:

- Complete Blood Count (CBC)—May show a mild to moderate leukocytosis with a shift to the left and a decreased hemoglobin and hematocrit, if previous bleeding has occurred.
- Urinalysis—WBC or RBC or bacteriuria may be present if there is a colovesical fistula.
- Blood Cultures—Should be obtained before parental antibiotics are initiated.

Plain X-ray films of the abdomen may be the initial study. Gas in the bowel wall may be seen in acute diverticulitis. Upright and lateral views can show free air within the peritoneal cavity as air under the diaphragm or air under the abdominal wall (Oeffinger, 2000).

Computerized tomography (CT) of the abdomen is the test of choice for immediate confirmation of acute diverticulitis (Goroll & Mulley, 2000). Inflammation of the pericolic tissue, presence of a single diverticulum or multiple diverticula, abscesses, and thickening of the bowel wall can be detected. Advantages of this imaging method are the relative noninvasiveness, the ability to visualize the bowel wall and pericolonic tissues, and the ability to rule out other intra-abdominal pathologic conditions (Ferzoco, Raptopoulos, & Silen, 1998). CT guided percutaneous drainage of abscesses can also be performed if necessary.

Ultrasound is also used in diagnosing diverticulitis. The ultrasound shows the thickening of the colon wall and presence of diverticula. The disadvantage of the ultrasound is that it is technician dependent and adequate pressure may not be applied due to patient tenderness or pain. The ultrasound quality is also often poor in obese patients.

A barium enema contrast study is not used during an acute phase of diverticulitis related to the possibility of dislodging an obstructing fecalith and causing a perforation (Ferzoco, Raptopoulos, & Silen, 1998). A barium enema is sometimes used after the acute episode to determine the extent of the disease.

A flexible sigmoidoscopy and colonoscopy are also not recommended in the acute phase of diverticulitis related to the increase of intraluminal pressure and possible perforation.

The physician must also consider and rule out other similar conditions such as irritable bowel syndrome or ischemic colitis. Both produce similar signs and symptoms of mild, uncomplicated diverticulitis. Adenocarcinoma or volvulus of the sigmoid colon can present as complicated diverticulitis with obstruction. Crohn's disease or ulcerative colitis may look like acute diverticulitis with a fistula.

GENERAL NURSING CARE

For the client with a diagnosis of diverticular disease, nursing care focuses on client education to help prevent a case of diverticulitis. The nurse first explains diverticulosis and the possible complication of diverticulitis, emphasizing that presently there is no known connection of diverticular disease with a family history or any genetic issues and that diverticular disease is a disease that increases in incidence with age and is associated with a dietary intake low in fiber.

The nurse explains what dietary fiber is, the recommended daily allowance, why fiber is important and vital to maintain a healthy bowel, and how water intake is necessary for the fiber to be effective. (See chapter 10 for nutritional issues in the older adult.)

The nurse in collaboration with the dietitian obtains a dietary intake history, including allergies, food preferences, religious or personal food restrictions, and a 24–48 hour detail diet intake. With this information the nurse, dietitian, and client can begin to formulate a diet to meet daily requirements. Client education regarding regular bowel movements, preventing constipation and daily activity and exercise is also stressed by the nurse (Table 11.3).

Nursing care for the client with a diagnosis of mild to acute diverticulitis involves client education regarding the treatment plan, mainly bowel rest

TABLE 11.3   Nursing Care Plan for Diverticulosis in the Older Adult

Nursing Diagnosis	Client Outcome	Nursing Interventions
Altered nutrition: less than body requirements of fiber R/T knowledge deficit	• The client will have a daily dietary intake of 25–35 grams of fiber every day.	• Collect and assess dietary history, including: food allergies, preferences, religious or cultural restrictions, and a 24–28 hour diet recall. • Explain role of fiber in maintaining healthy bowel function. • Identify foods high in fiber (Table 11.8) • Discuss the role of fiber supplements. • Plan a diet with the client and dietitian that will include the daily requirements of fiber using food sources and fiber supplements.
Risk for fluid volume deficit R/T increased vulnerability secondary to decreased fluid reserve and decreased sensation of thirst.	• The client will maintain adequate fluid intake of 8–10 eight-ounce glasses of water every day (unless contraindicated).	• Assess the client's daily intake of water. • Teach the client the relationship of water intake to fiber in order for fiber to be effective. • Explain the role of water in maintaining moist stool to prevent constipation. • Assist the client to set up a regular schedule for fluid intake.
Risk for constipation	• The client will demonstrate improved bowel elimination: soft brown stool every 1 to 3 days.	• Assess potential contributing factors such as bowel schedule, exercise, diet/fluid intake. • Discuss and plan with the client a regular time for defecation as part of daily routine. • Encourage daily walking to maintain abdominal muscle tone (unless contraindicated).
Knowledge Deficit: signs and symptoms of diverticulitis	• The client will verbalize the signs and symptoms of diverticulitis.	• Explain the progression from diverticulosis to diverticulitis: the inflammation process, a fecal plug in a diverticulum, possible abscess or perforation of the intestines.

(continued)

TABLE 11.3 *(continued)*

Nursing Diagnosis	Client Outcome	Nursing Interventions
		• Teach the signs and symptoms of diverticulitis: fever, LLQ pain, nausea, and vomiting • Explain importance of early reporting of signs and symptoms to the primary health care provider or going to the emergency department. • Teach the rationale for changing to a low-fiber diet during episodes of diverticulitis. Give list of low-fiber foods and plan a low-fiber diet within the primary care provider's guidelines.

(clear liquids or NPO), antibiotic medications for the inflammation, pain control, and alleviation of signs and symptoms (Table 11.4).

For the client with severe diverticulitis requiring surgery, nursing care focuses on the usual preoperative patient education, coughing, deep breathing, turning, ambulation, nasogastric tube, TED stockings, pain management, foley catheter, and in addition teaching about a colostomy (purpose) and stoma marking. The stoma marking is usually done by an enterostomal therapy (ET) nurse (Table 11.5). Because of the risk of bowel perforation, aggressive bowel preparation is usually not prescribed.

The postoperative nursing care and client teaching for a bowel resection procedure, with or without a colostomy, are like other major abdominal surgeries. The nursing care focuses on providing pain relief and preventing postoperative complications. Nursing interventions focus on turning, coughing, deep breathing, use of an incentive spirometer, leg exercises, and increasing mobility and out-of-bed activities. The nurse also assesses the surgical incision and colostomy, if applicable, for any signs of infection or vascular compromise.

In addition to the care and interventions just mentioned, the nurse must assess the older adult client critically, looking for any subtle signs and symptoms of postoperative complications. The older adult client may not have an increase in temperature or an increase in the WBC, even in the presence of an infection. The nurse is also vigilant in assessing the incision

TABLE 11.4 Nursing Care Plan for Mild to Acute Diverticulitis

Nursing Diagnosis	Client Outcome	Nursing Intervention
Pain R/T inflammation of diverticulum.	• The client will verbalize a decrease in pain.	• Assess the client's pain: exact location, quality, quantity, client's goal for pain relief. • Provide pain relief with prescribed analgesics (Demerol drug of choice). • Initiate antibiotics as prescribed immediately after blood cultures are drawn.
Risk for increasing inflammation	• The client will demonstrate: temperature less than 101°F and WBC below 10,000 mm³. • The client will verbalize a decrease in pain. • The client will verbalize the signs and symptoms to immediately report to the primary care provider.	Outpatient • Explain importance of bowel rest and the need for a clear liquid diet. • Teach proper administration of antibiotics: take on time, take until end of prescribed course, food/medication interactions. • Teach signs and symptoms to report immediately: temperature continues to be elevated, unrelieved pain or increasing intensity, any nausea and vomiting, any rectal bleeding. Inpatient • Monitor temperature every four hours. • Assess WBC with each laboratory order. • Assess abdomen every four hours: Auscultate bowel sounds, palpate for tenderness and masses especially LLQ, assess for distention, if NG tube present: assess placement and drainage. • Assess for pain relief from analgesic. • Initiate parental IV antibiotics • Assess hydration status: I&O maintain IV fluids, B/P & P.

TABLE 11.5   Nursing Care Plan for Severe Diverticulitis (Surgery)

Nursing Diagnosis	Client Outcome	Nursing Interventions
Knowledge deficit: pre-operative teaching	• The client will demonstrate/verbalize understanding of: coughing and deep breathing, use of incentive spirometer, leg exercises, turning every 2 to 4 hours, need for N/G tube, IV fluids, foley catheter, and dressing changes, potential for colostomy.	• Discuss with the client the rationale for postoperative activities and exercises. • Demonstrate deep breathing, coughing, incentive spirometer, leg exercises, turning, and position. • Discuss the need of NPO status, IV fluids, NG tube, and dressings. • Discuss and explain the role of the enterostomal therapist and the potential need for colostomy and marking the location of the colostomy before surgery.
Risk for postoperative complications R/T impaired mobility secondary to abdominal surgery and pain.	• The client will not develop post operative complications such as: atelectasis, ileus, deep vein thrombosis.	• Turn and reposition every 2 hours for the first 24 hours and then every 4 hours & prn, encourage leg exercises, assist client to use the incentive spirometer, cough & deep breath every 2 hours for the first 24 hours post-op, and then every 4 hours while awake until discharge.
Management of therapeutic regimen, effective: individual	• The client will verbalize rationale for gradually increasing dietary intake of fiber and adequate intake of water. • The client will relate the importance of a regular bowel elimination regimen such as not ignoring the urge to defecate and not straining for a bowel movement. • The client will relate the importance of moderate activity and exercise in maintaining effective bowel function.	• Explain/reinforce the rationale for 25–35 grams of fiber every day to maintain healthy bowel function. • Explain and plan a slow increase in adding fiber to the diet to prevent bloating and/or gas. • Explain the role of fiber supplements and avoiding harsh laxatives. • Explain/reinforce the importance of adequate water intake to keep the stool soft and moist so that the stool will move through the bowel easily.

TABLE 11.5 *(continued)*

Nursing Diagnosis	Client Outcome	Nursing Interventions
Body image disturbance R/T formation of colostomy.	• The client will verbalize and demonstrate acceptance of appearance of colostomy. • The client will demonstrate a willingness to perform colostomy care.	• Establish a therapeutic relationship by: encouraging the client to express feeling regarding ostomy and bowel functioning, acknowledge the client's feelings, encourage questions regarding care and prognosis, clarify misinformation and provide reliable information about ostomy care and functioning. • Prepare family for physical and emotional changes, support the family. • Assist the client to accept help from others. • Provide opportunity to share with other people who are experiencing similar situations. • Begin to gradually incorporate the client in the care of the ostomy and appliance.

because wound healing may be slower in the older adult and skin may break down faster.

NURSING DIAGNOSES AND PLAN OF CARE

Review Tables 11.3, 11.4, and 11.5.

INTERVENTIONS, TREATMENTS, ALTERNATIVE TREATMENTS

Medical Intervention and Treatment

For many older adults, diverticulitis is treated on an outpatient basis. This is the client who presents with a mild, uncomplicated case without systemic signs and symptoms, is able to understand and follow the treatment plan, and can take oral fluids and oral medications. The treatment plan usually consists of clear liquids to provide the bowel with rest, a broad spectrum antibiotic sensitive to gram-negative enteric aerobes (e.g., trimethoprim-sulfamethoxazole or ciprofloxacin or cephalexin), and an antibiotic effective against anaerobes (metromidazole or clindamycin), both taken for 7 to 10 days (see Table 11.6). Strong opiate analgesics and antipyretics are not prescribed in order to not mask signs of increasing inflammation. The client is instructed on signs and symptoms to report to the physician or to go to the emergency department. These signs and symptoms are increase in fever over 101°F, increase in pain, or the inability to drink fluids. Improvement is expected within 48 hours. When the pain has stopped, a slow progression back to a low residue diet may start. If improvement is not achieved, the client is admitted for inpatient treatment and further evaluation.

Hospitalization is recommended for increasing pain, fever, or inability to take oral fluids and medication, and for older adults who may not present some of the classic signs and symptoms, such as the immunocompromised or clients taking steroids. The inpatient treatment consists of nothing by mouth, a nasogastric (NG) tube if small bowel distention or obstruction is present, intravenous fluids, parental antibiotics, and an analgesic for pain, if needed. Meperidol (Demerol) is the drug of choice for pain associated with diverticulitis. Morphine is not recommended because it can increase segmentation and intraluminal pressure. The standard acute triple antibiotic therapy is intravenous ampicillin, an aminoglycoside, and metronidazole (Freeman, 2001) (Table 11.6). Again improvement, decreased pain, decreased fever, and decreased leukocytosis is expected within 48 hours. If signs and symptoms continue this may indicate an unresolved abscess. A CT scan will be needed to evaluate the effectiveness or ineffectiveness of the medical treatment and if an abscess requires percutaneous drainage.

If improvement is noted, the client is advanced to a clear liquid diet progressing to a low residue diet. Six to eight weeks after resolution, the client is evaluated with a colonoscopy. If there is no improvement after 48 hours, then surgery becomes the treatment of choice.

A client presenting with signs and symptoms of free perforation with either purulent or fecal peritonitis or a patient with sepsis from an undrainable abscess or unrelieved low bowel obstruction, requires medical support and surgical exploration (www.fascrs.org/coresubjects/2001/young-fadok). Medical support consists of nothing by mouth (possible NG tube), intrave-

TABLE 11.6   Common Medications Used to Treat Diverticular Disease

Medication	Nursing Implications	Client Teaching
Trimethoprim-sulfamethoxazole (Bactrim, Septra, Septra DS)	• Precautions with clients with renal disease, elderly. Impaired hepatic/renal function, bronchial asthma. • I&O, assess BUN, creatinine. • Assess for blood dyscrasias, skin rash, sore throat, bruising, bleeding, fatigue, joint pain.	• Take each oral dose with a full 8 ounce glass of water. • Take on an empty stomach, 1 hour before a meal or 2 hours after a meal. • Complete full course of medication. • Avoid sunlight or use sunscreen. • Avoid over the counter (OTC) medications, aspirin and vitamin C unless directed by the physician. • Notify physician if skin rash, sore throat, fever, mouth sores, unusual bruising, bleeding occur.
Ciprofloxacin (Cipro)	• Assess kidney and liver function studies. • I&O. • Administer 2 hours before or after antacids, zinc, iron, calcium.	• Do not take any products containing magnesium, calcium, iron, or aluminum with this drug or within 2 hours of the drug. • Complete full course of medication. • Increase fluid intake to 3 liters (3 quarts) a day. • Avoid sunlight or use sunscreen. • Do not take theophylline with this drug.
Cephalexin (Keflex)	• Assess for sensitivity to penicillin and other cephalosporins. • Nephrotoxicity: increased BUN, creatinine, I&O. • Assess liver function tests. • Assess bowel function: diarrhea • Anaphylaxis signs & symptoms may occur a few days after therapy begins	• Do not drink alcohol while taking medication. • Use yogurt or buttermilk to decrease potential diarrhea. • Complete full course of medication.

(continued)

TABLE 11.6 (continued)

Medication	Nursing Implications	Client Teaching
Metornidida-zole (Flagyl)	• I&O, weigh daily. • Assess stools for amount, consistency, and color. • Neurotoxicity.	• Do not drink alcohol while taking. • Urine may turn dark reddish-brown. • May have a metallic taste. • Notify physician for numbness or tingling of extremities. • Complete full course of medication.
Clindamycin (Cleocin)	• Assess blood studies: liver enzymes, WBC, RBC, Hct & Hgb, iron, reticulocytes. • Assess for psuedomembranous colitis. • Take with 8 ounces of water. • Assess respiratory status.	• Take with a full 8-ounce glass of water. • May take with food. • Complete course of medication. • Do not break, crush, or chew capsule. • Report sore throat, fever, fatigue, diarrhea to physician. • Take medication at equal intervals around the clock.
Ampicillin (IV)	• May dilute in 50 mL, given over 10–15 minutes. • Assess for penicillin allergy. • Nephrotoxic, especially with a compromised renal system. • I&O, hematuria, oliguria. • Assess liver studies (AST, ALT), renal studies (Bun, creatinine, protein, blood), blood studies (WBC, RBC, Hgb, Hct, bleeding time). • Skin eruptions up to 1 week after discontinuing drug.	• Report sore throat, fever, fatigue, diarrhea, rash.

TABLE 11.6 *(continued)*

Medication	Nursing Implications	Client Teaching
Gentamicin (IV) (aminoglycoside)	• Give in 3 equally divided doses, dilute in 25 to 200 mL and give over 30–60 minutes. • Accurate weight, dose calculated per weight. • Nephrotoxic especially with a compromised renal system. • Assess renal studies (Bun, creatinine, protein, blood), I&O, fluids of 2–3 liters/day (unless contraindicated). • Ototoxicity, assess for ringing in ears, vertigo. • During infusion, assess for hypotension and assess pulse rate. • Assess IV site for thrombophlebitis. • Consult with physician regarding peak blood levels.	• Report headache, dizziness, symptoms of other infections (perineal itching, diarrhea, sores in mouth, changes in cough or sputum). • Report any hearing loss, ringing in ears, or feeling of fullness in head.
Metronidazole IV (Flagyl IV)	• Accurate weight, dose weight determined. • Give diluted dose over 1 hour or more. • Store in light resistant container, do not refrigerate. • Contraindicated: renal disease, hepatic disease, contracted visual or color fields, blood dyscrasias, CNS disorders. • Neurotoxicity: peripheral neuropathy, seizures, dizziness, uncoordination, pruritis, joint pains. • Superinfection: fever, monilial growth, fatigue, malaise.	• Urine may turn dark reddish-brown. • May cause metallic taste. • Report any numbness or tingling of extremities.

Adapted from: Skidmore-Roth, 2002.

nous hydration, electrolyte replacement, pain management, oxygenation and preparation for surgery with patient consent, and stoma marking. Stoma marking is done preoperatively except in rare emergency cases. The marking ensures that the stoma will be positioned correctly. The ET nurse assesses the contours, bony features and scars of the abdomen as well as the eyesight and manual dexterity of the client. It is important that the stoma be positioned so that the client can care for it easily.

Surgery may also be the outcome for the older adult who was initially diagnosed as acute or complicated and the client's condition continues to deteriorate. This could be indicated by increasing pain, more localized peritonitis, diffuse tenderness, increasing WBC, or if drainage of the abscess has not caused an improvement in the client's condition.

There are four basic surgical options: 1) primary resection with anastomosis, 2) primary resection, anastomosis, and proximal stoma, 3) 2-stage colostomy and resection (Hartmann procedure), and 4) 3-stage colostomy and drainage only (www.fascrs.org/coresubjects/2001/young-fadok). The primary resection with anastomosis is the procedure of choice when a client undergoes elective operative therapy after successful medical management and/or abscesses are adequately drained by percutaneous means (Ferzoco, Raptopoulos, & Silen, 1998). The client's condition must be stable and bowel ends healthy and nonedematous. Current trends include the laporoscopic approach to this sigmoid resection (Ferzoco, Raptopoulos, & Silen, 1998). Laparoscopy is safe and effective and usually leads to a faster recovery and shorter stay than conventional open surgery.

The two-stage primary resection, anastomosis, and proximal stoma resects the diseased colon, creates a primary anastomosis and creates a proximal diverting loop colostomy or loop ileostomy. The loop ileostomy or colostomy is reversed when the anastomosis has healed.

The two-stage colostomy and resection (Hartmann procedure) removes the diseased colon, creates a colostomy, and staples the rectal stump. After the rectal stump has healed and the infection has resolved, the colostomy is reversed and anastomosed to the rectal stump.

The three-stage transverse colostomy and drainage procedure first provides for drainage of abscesses and gross fecal peritonitis and creates a transverse colostomy. The second stage is removing the diseased segment of the colon and creating a colostomy. The third stage is the colostomy reversal. This procedure has a high morbidity and mortality (Ferzoco, Raptopoulos, & Silen, 1998) and has essentially been eliminated except for rare, unusual circumstances.

HEALTH PROMOTION AND QUALITY OF LIFE ISSUES

The key to health promotion for diverticular disease is prevention. This means preventing diverticulosis and preventing diverticulosis from becoming diverticulitis. One way to do this is through education. As one ages the presence of diverticula increases. It is a part of normal aging. Diverticulosis is a disease state that can go unnoticed without signs and symptoms until an acute attack of diverticulosis occurs. Therefore educating health care providers and older adults about the causal relationship of a diet low in fiber and diverticulosis is the first step. In the United States our fast food mentality and the increase of processed foods has significantly reduced the amount of fiber intake. Fiber, which was once called roughage, comes from plants. Whole grains, fruits, and vegetables are the most common sources of fiber in the diet. Fiber cannot be digested by saliva, or the enzymes in the stomach. Fiber goes into the intestines as fiber. Fiber is essential for healthy intestinal tract function. Fiber helps prevent not cure many intestinal dysfunctions. The American Dietetic Association recommends 20–35 grams of fiber each day. Table 11.7 lists some common foods and their fiber content. When instructing about increasing fiber intake, the nurse also cautions the client to begin adding fiber to the diet gradually in order to prevent bloating and flatus.

If the client is unable to take in sufficient amounts of fiber by diet, a bulk forming supplement may also be prescribed, such as Citrucel or Metamucil. These products are mixed with water and provide 4–6 grams of fiber. In the past physicians suggested avoiding "irritating foods" such as foods with small seeds, grape skins, corn or nuts. This is now a controversial point with no evidence to support it. Many physicians now prescribe a high-fiber diet without insisting on any dietary restrictions

The second step is teaching the importance of drinking eight to ten 8-ounce glasses of water each day, explaining how the fiber absorbs the water and makes the stool mass moist and soft so that it movers easier and faster through the bowel. This helps prevent constipation and decreases the need to strain at having a bowel movement. Unless fluid restrictions are part of the health care plan of the older adult, the water intake is essential when any oral bulking agent is used. If the tablet form of bulking agent is used, water intake is critically important.

The third step is teaching the signs and symptoms of diverticulitis and explaining how important it is to seek medical help immediately if the signs and symptoms occur. When teaching the older adult it is also important to

TABLE 11.7   Food Sources for Fiber

FRUITS				VEGETABLES	
Apples	1 = 5.8 grams	Brussels sprouts	1/2 cup = 3.4 grams	Romaine lettuce	1 cup = 1.0 grams
Oranges	1 = 3.1 grams	Cabbage	1/2 cup = 0.4 grams	Spinach	1/2 cup = 0.7 grams
Peaches	1 = 1.4 grams	Carrots	1 = 2.3 grams	Corn	1/2 cup = 2.0 grams
Strawberries	1/2 cup = 1.9 grams	Potatoes, peeled	1 = 1.8 grams	Green beans	1/2 cup = 1.0 grams
Blueberries	1/2 cup = 1.4 grams	Tomatoes	1 = 1.6 grams	Zucchini	1 cup = 0.6 grams
Raspberries	1/2 cup = 2.9 grams	Asparagus	1/2 cup = 0.7 grams		
Grapes	10 = 0.4 grams	Broccoli	1/2 cup = 1.2 grams		
Bananas	1 = 1.8 grams	Cauliflower	1/2 cup = 1.2 grams		

STARCHY VEGETABLES				GRAINS	
Lima beans	1/2 cup = 2.9 grams	Brown rice	1 cup = 2.0 grams	Raisin bran	1 cup = 4.0 grams
Kidney beans	1/2 cup = 3.2 grams	White rice	1 cup = 1.3 grams	All bran	1/3 cup = 10.0 grams
Navy beans	1/2 cup = 3.3 grams	Cooked oats	2/3 cup = 2.7 grams	Bran buds	1/3 cup = 8.0 grams
Lentils	1/2 cup = 4.0 grams	Whole wheat bread	1 slice = 2.0 grams		

Adapted from: Netzer, 1992.

stress that the usual signs and symptoms may not always be present in an older adult. Emphasizing that diffuse abdominal pain or mental confusion or fatigue, even without a fever, is sufficient to seek medical help.

The older adult may have diverticulosis, be symptom free, and not know he/she has the disease. In this case, the quality of life would not be influenced by this disease. By preventing diverticulitis quality of life can be maintained. Preventing pain and suffering from an acute attack of diverticulitis can allow the client to continue with ADLs, to socialize with family and friends, and to continue with hope and plans for the future.

If surgery is required for treatment of the diverticulitis, the potential for a colostomy, either temporary or permanent is great. Many people have difficulty accepting this altered bowel elimination pattern. Many patients find it difficult and embarrassing to talk about and to care for the colostomy. The client may be embarrassed about the potential for malodor or accidental leakage of stool. This may hinder socialization with others or even prevent the client from wanting to leave home for groceries, church, or even physician visits.

HOME MANAGEMENT AND SELF-CARE ISSUES

It is important to give the adult client both verbal and written instructions. As stated earlier, client education regarding diet, fluids, bowel movements, and activity should be included. If the client had surgery, additional information regarding signs and symptoms of wound infection and postoperative complications would also be included. If the client required a colostomy, additional instructions and supplies would be given as well as a referral for home health support and an ET nurse.

In addition to this teaching with the older adult client, the nurse must assess and evaluate the physical abilities and other health conditions of the client, such as:

Diet: When assessing and planning potential diet changes, the nurse must also assess the client's ability to chew foods thoroughly and the client's ability to swallow effectively. If the client has no teeth, no dentures, or improper fitting dentures, the client is likely to eat only liquids and soft foods, foods low in fiber. If the client has a swallowing impairment, again the client is likely to eat only liquids and soft foods.

Fluids: Teaching the client to increase fluid (water) intake may not be effective if the client has stress incontinence for example, and the way the client copes with the incontinence is to limit the intake of fluids (water).

Bowel Movements: The older adult experiences aging changes that slow down peristalsis and may result in less frequent bowel movements. However the advertising media frequently emphasize taking laxatives to promote daily bowel movements. Most of these ads target the older adult. Special emphasis on explaining the difference between bulk-forming supplements and actual laxatives or enemas is a high priority for the nurse.

Activity: For all clients, education regarding bending and straining is important. For the older adult client, assessment of living quarters will help the nurse understand how much "bending, reaching, and straining" the client may do each day. The nurse can recommend that the client store frequently used items at a level above the knees and below the shoulders, in order to avoid unnecessary strain or bending.

The older adult client may also have physical limitations and decreased energy. These could also be contributing factors to diet choices. It is easier to open a can of soup or use processed foods that are easy to prepare than to peel and clean fresh vegetables.

Another consideration for self-care issues is the financial resources of the client. Frequently the older adult may be on a fixed income. Fresh fruits and vegetables (good fiber sources) are expensive and may be unrealistic for the older adult client.

FOLLOW-UP CARE

The client is encouraged to make regular follow up visits with the physician. Frequently a referral to a gastroenterologist after an acute episode of diverticulitis is indicated. After the client has responded to treatment and the signs and symptoms of diverticulitis have subsided, a colonoscopy is usually performed to evaluate the colon and the extent of the disease. The colonoscopy can also help rule out any other colon diseases.

Even with medical intervention, symptoms will return in approximately one-third of all patients treated for diverticulitis (Dunphy & Winland-Brown, 2001). It is important to help clients understand that even if they adhere to the proper diet, fluids, and medications, that they may have another attack of diverticulitis. Therefore it is important to follow up with the primary health care provider if they develop any signs and symptoms of diverticulitis or infection.

CONCLUSION

Diverticulosis of the colon is a disease that mainly affects the older adult. The increase in prevalence is thought to be due to the decrease in fiber intake seen in the industrialized world. However, about 70% of older adults with diverticulosis are either asymptomatic or have infrequent symptoms and rarely seek medical attention. Symptomatic diverticulosis requires examination to rule out colon cancer. When diverticulitis occurs, management should include fluid replacement and bowel rest. Treatment with antibiotics is commonplace and they should be taken for the entire length of the prescribed therapy.

With dietary changes and control of acute episodes, diverticular disease can be controlled successfully and the older adult can return to activities of daily living without restrictions.

REFERENCES

Bilhartz, L. E., & Croft, C. L. (2000). *Gastrointestinal disease in primary care.* Philadelphia: Lippincott Williams & Wilkins.

Deckmann, R. C., & Cheskin, L. J. (1993). Diverticular disease in the elderly. *Journal of American Geriatric Society, 41*(9), 986–993.

Dunphy, L. M., & Winland-Brown, J. E. (2001). *Primary care: The art and science of advanced practice nursing.* Philadelphia: F. A. Davis.

Ferzoco, L. B., Raptopoulos, V., & Silen, W. (1998). Acute diverticulitis. *The New England Journal of Medicine, 338*(21), 1521–1526.

Freeman, S. R. (2001). Diverticulitis. In P. R. McNally (Ed.), *GI/Liver secrets* (pp. 357–363). Philadelphia: Hanley & Belfus, Inc.

http://www.fascrs.org/coresubjects/2001/young-fadok.html

Mirsha, G. (2002). Diverticular disease of the colon. *Emergency Medicine, 34*(2), 66.

Netzer, C. T. (1992). *Encyclopedia of food values.* New York: Dell.

National Digestive Diseases Information Clearinghouse (1991, October). *Diverticulosis and diverticulitis.* NIH Publication 92-1163. Washington, DC: Author.

National Digestive Diseases Information Clearinghouse (1986, August). *Digestive health and disease: A Glossary.* NIH Publication 86-2750. Washington, DC: Author.

Oeffinger, K. C. (2000). Diverticulitis. In L. E. Bilhartz & C. L. Croft (Eds.), *Gastrointestinal disease in primary care* (pp. 164–174). Philadelphia: Lippincott Williams & Wilkins.

Skidmore-Roth, L. (2002). *Mosby's nursing drug reference.* St. Louis: Mosby.

−12−

Constipation and Noninfectious Diarrhea

Lynn Ferebee and Sue E. Meiner

Constipation and noninfectious diarrhea are two abnormal conditions of bowel elimination. Each will be addressed individually.

Constipation is a health issue that will affect everyone at least once during his or her lifetime. The effects of constipation can be a temporary inconvenience or severe enough to greatly impact the person's quality of life. Approximately twelve percent of adults use laxatives routinely (Norton, 1996). Contrary to popular belief, the incidence of constipation does not become more prevalent with advancing age (Abyad, 1998). Estimates of the prevalence of constipation among older adults vary according to the definition used. Over half of the elderly who complain of constipation move their bowels at least once daily. In one study, 47% of interview respondents reported constipation, but only 17% had two or fewer bowel movements per week (Harari, 1999). The frequency of bowel movements in healthy older adults is nearly the same as in younger persons. Nevertheless, the use of laxatives is more common among older adults, even when stools are fairly frequent (Harari, 1999). Following the definition of constipation, a review of pathophysiology and factors that contribute to constipation, patient assessment with diagnostic testing, and suggested nursing interventions will be presented. Then noninfectious diarrhea will be defined, a review of pathophysiology and factors that contribute to diarrhea, patient assessment with diagnostic testing and appropriate nursing interventions will follow.

CONSTIPATION

Constipation is not easily defined. The patient's definition of constipation is not always congruent with the medical definition of constipation. The Mosby's Medical, Nursing, & Allied Health Dictionary (1998) defines constipation as a condition in which bowel movements are not regular, the feces are hard and small, or bowel movements are difficult or painful. The frequency of bowel movements may vary considerably from person to person and what is normal cannot be precisely defined. Many older adults equate good health with daily bowel movements (Imershein & Linnehan, 2000). Simple constipation is often related to lifestyle. The patient avoids or postpones bowel movements to a more convenient time (Storrie, 1997). Idiopathic slow constipation refers to fewer bowel movements and the patient experiences pain and bloating (Storrie, 1997). Outlet obstruction, paradoxical contraction, or anismus all refer to the patient's inability to relax the external anal sphincter muscle during defecation despite straining (Storrie, 1997). Weak pelvic floor and descending perineum syndrome is the result of nerve damage during childbirth or excessive straining during bowel movements over a prolonged period of time (Storrie, 1997). Weak rectovaginal septum is the condition of a rectocele greater than three centimeters and rectal emptying is difficult (Storrie, 1997).

ETIOLOGY

Hypoactivity of the colon is one cause of constipation. Specific drug categories that contribute to constipation include opiates, antichlonergics, antidepressants, and calcium or aluminum antacids (Sodeman & Haider, 1998). Eating disorders, hypokalemia, and dehydration also contribute to hypoactivity of the colon (Kidd & Robinson, 2000). Factors such as immobility, reduced fiber in the diet, and reduced oral intake all contribute to constipation. The physical influences of colorectal lesions and tumors are direct physical causes of constipation (Sodeman & Haider, 1998). Difficulty passing the stool due to hard consistency, hemorrhoids, rectal fissures, rectal ulcers, rectocele, incompetent pelvic floor, paradoxical pelvic floor contractions, ineffective abdominal effort, inadequate bathroom facilities, neuropathy, or a confused mental state also may result in constipation (Norton, 1996). If a person does not respond to the immediate urge to defecate, this may contribute to constipation. The patient's perception may be altered due to the aging process (Imershein & Linnehan, 2000). Patients with constipation often complain of abdominal pain, cramping or bloating, and general malaise or fatigue. In severe cases of constipation, patients may experience nausea, headaches, and halitosis (Norton, 1996). Anorexia, overflow diarrhea, confusion, nausea, vomiting, or urinary dysfunctions are also common patient complaints of discomfort (Fallon & O'Neill, 1997). See Table 12.1 for a listing of the contributing factors for bowel hypoactivity.

PATHOPHYSIOLOGY

Food is introduced to the mouth and is mechanically chewed and swallowed and then passes through the esophagus and enters the stomach. The food is mixed with digestive juices and dwells in the stomach for several hours and becomes chyme. The peristaltic waves move the chyme through the pylorus into the first portion of the small intestine called the duodenum, then through the jejunum, and finally into the ileum. The primary function of the small intestine is fat and protein digestion and absorption. The ileocecal separates the small intestines from the large intestines, which consist of the cecum, appendix, ascending, transverse, descending, sigmoid colon, and finally the rectum. The large intestine is approximately 1.5 meters in length. As the 500 to 700 cc of chyme passes into the large intestines, it is now considered fecal material. The fecal mass is passed through the colon with segmental colonic movements during the fasting

TABLE 12.1   Contributing Factors for Hypoactivity of the Bowel

1. Inadequate dietary fiber
2. Immobility
3. Neuropathy
4. Hormonal or endocrine disorders
5. Medications
6. Diseases of the colon
7. Psychiatric disorders

Adapted from: Norton, C. (1996). The causes and nursing management of constipation. *British Journal of Nursing, 5*,(20), 1252–1258.

phase of the gut. Absorption of water and electrolytes occur during this phase. The extrinsic and intrinsic autonomic nerve and intestinal hormones determine the rate of the gastrointestinal functions. When the rectum becomes distended with the fecal mass, the urge to defecate is stimulated. When defecation occurs the external sphincter relaxes (McCance & Huether, 1998).

At approximately fifty years of age the body starts the phase of the aging process characterized by a decline in the senses of taste and smell. Poor fitting dentures contribute to changes in diet. Salivary secretions may decrease, which result in a dry mouth. Esophageal and gastric motility are diminished, as well as the volume and acid content of the gastric secretions (McCance & Huether, 1998).

Constipation is often the result of lifestyle variables rather than physiologic decline. Contributing causes of constipation include lifelong bowel habits, current diet, decreased oral intake, and decreased physical activity (McCance & Huether, 1998). The lifestyle variables may include little if any exercise or walking, i.e., a sedentary life. Some older adults start using laxatives regularly, with or without enemas, after a few bouts of constipation occur in late middle-age.

ASSESSMENT

During the patient assessment, it is important to obtain an accurate history (Abyad, 1998). Patient questions regarding stool frequency and stool consistency are crucial to the history (Fallon & O'Neill, 1997). Physical symptoms such as abdominal pain, abdominal bloating, and rectal bleeding should be verified (Abyad, 1998). Questions regarding laxative use and results should be discussed. Other factors to be evaluated include diet, oral fluid intake, exercise habits, sleep patterns, bathroom privacy, recent illnesses, treatment and current medication regimen (Vickery, 1997). The patient's views regarding constipation and willingness to make changes in lifestyle should also be included (Vickery, 1997).

The physical exam includes an abdominal exam to assess for bowel sounds and abdominal masses. The rectal exam should include an anal scope to assess for anorectal lesion, anal fissures, fistula, strictures, and hemorrhoids. The sphincter tone and strength should also be evaluated, and the stool should be checked for occult blood (Abyad, 1998).

DIAGNOSTIC STUDIES

Successful treatment of constipation requires an individualized plan that addresses the identified causes, lifestyle issues, and patient preferences.

After the history and physical exam have been completed, the patient may be referred for endoscopy and radiographic evaluations to eliminate physical causes of constipation such as colon cancer (Abyad, 1998). Colonic transit and colonic motility studies evaluate constipation by utilizing radiopaque markers to determine the time involved to pass the markers through the colon. Abdominal X-rays are taken 5 to 7 days after ingesting the markers (Abyad, 1998).

NURSING DIAGNOSIS

Altered elimination patterns of primary or simple constipation are generally related to:

1. Inadequate fluid intake
2. Inadequate dietary fiber intake
3. Inadequate physical activity
4. Personal habits
5. Lack of privacy
6. Emotional status
7. Pain on defecation
8. Ignoring the urge to defecate
9. Diagnostic procedures
10. Weak abdominal musculature (Vickery, 1997).

Altered elimination patterns of secondary constipation are related to:

1. Colon cancer
2. Dehydration
3. Diabetes mellitus
4. Hypercalcemia
5. Hypokalemia
6. Hypothyroidism
7. Parkinson's disease
8. Stroke
9. Palpable mass
10. Neuromuscular or musculoskeletal impairment
11. Chronic obstructive lesions (Vickery, 1997).

Altered elimination patterns of iatrogenic constipation are related to:

1. Aluminum hydroxide containing antacids
2. Anticholinergics

3. Calcium channel blockers
4. Diuretics
5. Iron supplements
6. Narcotics (Vickery, 1997).

PLAN OF CARE

The plan of care should be individualized for each patient according to his/her lifestyle, attitudes, beliefs, and needs. Potential barriers to the plan of care should be identified and anticipated to assist the patient with a successful outcome (Sheehy & Hall, 1998). The goal of constipation management is to establish regular bowel response to the urge to defecate without the need for laxatives (Vickery, 1997).

The bowel basics include the following and ideally begin with a clean, nonimpacted bowel (Weeks, Hubbartt, & Michaels, 2000):

1. Physical exercise
2. Increase fiber intake
3. Increase fluid intake
4. Reestablish bowel habits with bowel retraining (Abayad, 1998)
5. Patient to sit in an upright position on the toilet
6. Ensure patient privacy in the bathroom
7. Medication management
8. Patient education (Cash & Glass, 1998)

INTERVENTIONS

Laxatives and enemas should not be a part of routine bowel management. Older adults that have used laxatives for years require education about the harmful effects on the bowel. When possible, interventions should be planned over several months. Keeping a bowel log will demonstrate the true frequency of bowel evacuation and other daily practices that can lead to a healthier elimination routine (Cotter & Strumpf, 2002).

Routine interventions should include the following:

1. Physical exercise daily
2. Increase fiber intake: A well-known fiber recipe of two cups of Kellogg's All Bran, two cups applesauce and one cup of prune juice

mixed well. Give 30 to 60 cc daily (Weeks, Hubbartt, & Michaels, 2000). Fiber should be introduced to the diet slowly to avoid abdominal pain or bloating and flatulence (Copeman, 1997). Fiber improves the colon transit time and reduces water absorption. These factors determine the consistency and softness of the stool (Norton, 1996).

3. Increase fluid intake to 1.5 to 2 liters per day
4. Attempt a bowel movement at the same time every day, ideally 15 minutes after a meal
5. Instruct the patient not to ignore the urge to defecate (Kidd & Robinson, 1999)
6. Patient to sit in an upright position on the toilet (Weeks, Hubbartt, & Michaels, 2000).
7. Ensure patient privacy in the bathroom.
8. Medication management: Bulk-forming agents should be utilized first and adequate hydration necessary to avoid obstruction. Appropriate choices are Metamucil, Citrucel, and Fibercon (Cash & Glass, 2000). This intervention is not ideal and pharmacological intervention should be utilized if the above interventions have failed (Kidd & Robinson, 1999).
9. Patient education should dispel myths and self-defined definitions of constipation. Reassure the patient that three bowel movements a week is considered within normal range (Abyad, 1998). Chronic laxative use may delay spontaneous bowel movements for 4 to 6 weeks (Cash & Glass, 2000).

Patient education is prepared as a unique experience for each older adult according to the needs and educational level of that person. See Table 12.2 for points to remember during patient teaching activities.

QUALITY OF LIFE ISSUES

In the United States, patient complaints of constipation account for approximately two million primary care visits annually. It is estimated that $7.5 million is spent on laxatives yearly (Nursing 2001, 2001). Constipation is a problem that can greatly impact the quality of life. The severity of symptoms ranges from halitosis and headaches, to bloating with abdominal pain (Norton, 1996).

TABLE 12.2   Points to Remember in Patient Education

1. Constipation affects almost everyone at one time or another
2. Many people think they are constipated when, in fact, their bowel movements are regular
3. The most common causes of constipation are poor diet and lack of exercise
4. Additional causes of constipation include medications, irritable bowel syndrome, abuse of laxatives, and specific diseases
5. A medical history and physical examination may be the only diagnostic tests needed before the primary care provider suggests treatment
6. In most cases, following these simple tips will help relieve symptoms and prevent recurrence of constipation:
    a. Eat a well-balanced, high-fiber diet that includes beans, bran, whole grains, fresh fruits, and vegetables
    b. Drink plenty of water/fluids
    c. Exercise regularly
    d. Set aside time after breakfast or dinner for undisturbed visits to the toilet
    e. Do not ignore the urge to have a bowel movement
    f. Understand that normal bowel habits vary
    g. Whenever a significant or prolonged change in bowel habits occurs, check with the primary care provider
7. Most people with mild constipation do not need laxatives. However, health care providers may recommend laxatives for a limited time for people with chronic constipation.

From: National Digestive Diseases Information Clearinghouse, 2002.

HOME MANAGEMENT AND SELF-CARE ISSUES

The key to home management is lifestyle modification, and changes and routines regarding diet and exercise should be maintained (Sweeney, 1997). Many elders experience a reduced thirst sensation and often need to be reminded to drink more fluids (Yen, 1995). Older adults with constipation should avoid alcoholic drinks as well as beverages such as grapefruit juice, coffee, tea, colas, and chocolate (Weeks, Hubbartt, & Michaels, 2000). Medications taken by the patient should be evaluated for side effects of constipation. Patients may track bowel movements by marking a calendar. It is imperative to avoid bowel obstructions and dependence on laxatives.

NONINFECTIOUS DIARRHEA

Diarrhea can be either acute or chronic. The acute type usually lasts less than three weeks and is most often related to bacterial, viral, or parasitic infection. Chronic diarrhea lasts longer than three weeks and is usually related to a functional disorder. Two major functional disorders are irritable bowel syndrome (IBS), or inflammatory bowel disease. See chapter 11, for information on IBS. Inflammatory bowel disease is not presented in this book due to its length of presentation.

Noninfectious diarrhea may be accompanied by cramping, abdominal pain, bloating, and an urgent need to use the bathroom. Diarrhea can cause dehydration, which means the body lacks enough fluid to function properly. The frail elderly are especially vulnerable and treatment is needed promptly. See Table 12.3 for a list of the general signs of dehydration from diarrhea.

ETIOLOGY

Diarrhea can be caused by many factors such as a change in routine or diet, medications, surgery, or radiation treatments. Food intolerances are a common cause of diarrhea. Some people are unable to digest a component of food, such as lactose. The use of antibiotics can lead to the elimination of the needed flora in the intestinal tract, thus preventing proper digestion of foodstuffs and a rapid passing of food waste products. Certain blood pressure medications cause a rapid emptying of the GI tract and the use of antacids containing magnesium can lead to diarrhea.

PATHOLOGY

Chronic diarrhea can be subdivided into three categories: osmotic, secretory, and inflammatory. People with osmotic diarrhea usually have large amounts of undigested fat in the stool (steatorrhea). The condition is

TABLE 12.3 General Signs of Dehydration From Noninfectious Diarrhea

- Thirst
- Less frequent urination
- Dry skin
- Fatigue
- Light-headedness
- Dark colored urine

From: National Digestive Diseases Information Clearinghouse, 2002.

caused either by ingestion of poorly absorbed substances (magnesium or aluminum salts, or other oral laxatives), or by incomplete digestion and malabsorption of some food components. People with advanced chronic pancreatitis can lose the ability to digest dietary fat, which can lead to steatorrhea. Persons with bile duct obstruction or decreased bile production resulting from cirrhosis are unable to digest fat and can develop steatorrhea.

Secretory diarrhea usually results in large amounts of watery stool, ranging from two to five liters over a 24-hour period. It is caused by production and secretion of excessive fluid by the small intestine. Secretory diarrhea is usually caused by neuroendocrine tumors, which release hormones into the bloodstream that stimulate the small intestine to secrete excessive amounts of fluid and electrolytes.

Inflammatory changes in the bowel mucosa increase stool volume by decreasing the absorption of water from the stool, and can cause blood in the stool. This type of diarrhea is frequently seen with the diagnoses of Crohn's disease and ulcerative colitis.

GENERAL NURSING CARE

Patient education is essential regarding the rationale for avoiding the use of laxatives and cathartics, and selecting foods that provide nutrition with less fat and more fiber content. A bowel training program is recommended when chronic laxative abuse is involved. Toileting as a treatment option for frail elderly who are dependent for activities of daily living can be successful if the person is given the opportunity to evacuate at regular intervals.

Individually selected nursing actions may include recommending that the older adult cut down on solid foods for 24 to 48 hours, drink more fluids (sport electrolyte drinks like Gatorade may be helpful), take an antidiarrheal medication such as loperamide 2 mg tablets (Immodium), wash hands carefully, especially after using the toilet, and treat any rash and/or skin irritations around the anus with a recommended ointment. Instruction should include written material on ways to identify signs and symptoms of dehydration. Following treatment, if the diarrhea continues for more than 48 hours, contact with the primary care provider is essential (Zastocki & Rovinski-Wagner, 2000).

NURSING DIAGNOSES AND PLAN OF CARE

1. Diarrhea related to high stress levels and anxiety
    Definition: passage of loose unformed stools

Plan of Care: communicate with the patient until verbalization of understanding of the causative factors and rationale for treatment regimen including the reduction of stress (Doenges, Moorhouse & Geissler-Murr, 2000).

2. Coping, ineffective, related to inadequate level of confidence in ability to cope/perception of control
   Definition: inability to form a valid appraisal of the stressors, inadequate choices of practiced responses, and/or inability to use available resources.
   Plan of Care: assess current functional capacity and note how it is affecting the individual's coping ability; assess level of anxiety and coping on an ongoing basis (Doenges, Moorhouse & Geissler-Murr, 2000).

INTERVENTIONS AND TREATMENTS

Diagnostic tests can be ordered that will find the cause of chronic diarrhea. These tests include a stool culture to rule out infectious diarrhea, fasting tests to identify food intolerances or allergies. Sigmoidoscopy or colonoscopy may be needed to identify inflammatory conditions, polyps, diverticula, tumors, or other findings that could lead to a successful intervention plan.

Treatment is geared toward stopping the diarrhea and replacing the fluids and electrolytes as necessary. Until diarrhea subsides, avoiding milk products, greasy foods, and high-fiber or very sweet foods should be considered. These foods tend to aggravate diarrhea. As the diarrhea begins to subside and the cramping and bloating diminish, adding soft, bland foods to the diet is recommended. The foodstuffs that can be added include bananas, plain rice, boiled potatoes, toast, crackers, cooked carrots, and baked chicken without the skin or fat.

HEALTH PROMOTION AND QUALITY OF LIFE ISSUES

Eating a balanced diet with sufficient fiber and fluids to maintain hydration will promote a healthy GI tract. Regular physical activity is essential for sound motility of the GI tract and provides for a feeling of well-being. Avoiding the indiscriminate use of laxatives and cathartics, and making time for bowel evacuation on a regular basis is a healthy way to regain or maintain normal bowel functioning.

HOME MANAGEMENT AND SELF-CARE ISSUES

Most people with acute diarrhea can treat the symptoms with self-management and over-the-counter medications such as loperamide. Other antidiarrheal agents such as bismuth subsalicylate (Pepto-Bismol, Bismatrol), and kaolin or kaolin/pectin (Kaopectate, Kao-Spen, Kapectolin) can control noninfectious symptoms. It is vitally important that daily fluid intake be sufficient to combat dehydration.

FOLLOW-UP CARE

Follow-up care is indicated by the cause of the diarrhea. Usually ongoing monitoring is sufficient as long as fluid management is maintained and the symptoms do not change or continue beyond the expected recovery time frame.

CONCLUSION

Constipation is the most common gastrointestinal complaint in the United States, resulting in about two million annual visits to primary care providers. However, most people treat themselves without seeking medical attention. Although nearly everyone has an episode of constipation at some time, the incidence of constipation in older adults frequently is exaggerated. Keeping a diary of elimination for a two-week period just might provide the data that will help relieve the older adult of a preoccupation with bowel functioning. When true constipation is present, treatments can range from modifications in diet and fluid intake to medications. Frail elders with extremely limited mobility need close monitoring to prevent constipation. Health care providers need to be alert to the need for preventive measures and monitoring for all older adults.

Noninfectious diarrhea may be caused by allergies to food antigens in some older adults. Other causes may be functional bowel diseases. Overuse of laxatives is yet another potential cause for noninfectious diarrhea. Accurate diagnosis may be elusive. However, a sound medical history can guide an evaluation of chronic diarrhea. Detailed questioning about the characteristics of the stool is needed to determine the appropriate course of action. Even if the questions do not lead to a definitive diagnosis, symptomatic treatment with natural or synthetic opiates usually resolves the current episode. This will allow time to explore for the core cause of this often embarrassing health problem.

REFERENCES

Abyad, A. (1998). Constipation in the elderly: Diagnosis and management strategies. *Managed Care Interface*, 87–91.
Cash, J., & Glass, C. (2000). *Family practice guidelines*. Philadelphia: Lippincott.
Copeman, J. (1997). Advising older people on health dietary change. *Community Nurse*, 9, 16–17.
Cotter, V. T., & Strumpf, N. E. (2002). *Advanced practice nursing with older adults: Clinical guidelines* (pp. 208–212). Philadelphia: McGraw-Hill.
Doenges, M. E., Moorhouse, M. F., & Geissler-Murr, A. C. (2000). *Nurse's pocket guide: Diagnosis, interventions, and rationales* (8th ed.). Philadelphia: F. A. Davis Company.
Fallon, M., & O'Neill, B. (1997). ABC of palliative care: Constipation and diarrhoea. *British Medical Journal, 315*, 1293–1296.
Harari, D. (1999). Constipation in the elderly. In W. R. Hazzard, J. P. Blass, W. H. Ettinger, et al. (Eds.), *Principles of geriatric medicine and gerontology* (4th ed.). New York: McGraw-Hill.
Imershein, N., & Linnehan, E. (2000). Constipation: A common problem of the elderly. *Journal of Nutrition for the Elderly, 19*(3), 49–54.
Kidd, P., & Robinson, D. (1999). *Family nurse practitioner certification review*. St. Louis: Mosby.
McCance, K., & Huether, S. (1998). *Pathophysiology: The biologic basis for disease in adults and children* (3rd ed.). St. Louis: Mosby.
Mosby, (1998). *Mosby's medical, nursing & allied health dictionary* (5th ed.). St. Louis: The Company.
National Digestive Disease Information Clearinghouse (2002). Overview of digestive diseases. Available at *www.niddk.nih.gov/health/digest/pubs/overview.htm*
Norton, C. (1996). The causes and nursing management of constipation. *British Journal of Nursing, 5*(20), 1252–1258.
Nursing 2001 (2001). What you can do to prevent and treat constipation. *Nursing 2001 supplement: A guide to women's health*.
Sheehy, C., & Hall, G. R. (1998). Rethinking the obvious: A model for preventing constipation. *Journal of Gerontological Nursing, 24*(3), 38–44.
Sodeman, W., & Haider, K. (1998). Constipation in the nursing home patient. *Annual of Long-Term Care, 6*(2), 54–59.
Storrie, J. (1997). Biofeedback: A first-line treatment for idiopathic constipation. *British Journal of Nursing, 6*(3), 152–158.
Sweeney, M. (1997). Constipation: Diagnosis and treatment. *Home Care Provider, 2*(5), 250–255.
Vickery, G. (1997). Basics of constipation. *Gastroenterology Nursing, 20*(4), 125–128.
Weeks, S. K., Hubbartt, E., & Michaels, T. K. (2000). Keys to bowel success. *Rehabilitation Nursing, 25*(2), 66–69.
Yen, P. (1995). Digestive dilemmas. *Geriatric Nursing, 16*(3), 141–142.
Zastocki, D. K., & Rovinski-Wagner, C. (2000). *Home care: Patient and family instructions* (2nd ed.). Philadelphia: W. B. Saunders.

—13—

Hemorrhoids and Problems of the Anus and Rectum

Catherine Hill

Unlike symptoms of the upper digestive tract, problems of the anus and rectum have a distinctly private, even embarrassing, nature for some patients. Modesty, sexuality, and age on the part of patient and provider are significant influences on the incidence of perianal examinations (Borum, 1998). These influences also affect the frequency of symptom reporting. Bleeding, pain, and perianal itching are common presenting symptoms which many providers and patients mistakenly attribute to hemorrhoidal disease (Bilhartz & Croft, 2000). While cancer is the second most frequent diagnosis entertained, rectal prolapse, proctitis, and fecal impaction should also be considered. Perianal disorders are commonly underdiagnosed in the elderly for many reasons.

MODESTY, SEXUALITY, AND AGE

Many factors influence patients, physicians and nurses in the case finding, intervention, and teaching realms of anorectal disease. Some of these factors can be inferred from recent studies of 4,195 elderly Medicare patients in a preventive health study (Paglia, 1999), and 9,400 adults in the 1992 National Health Interview Study (Potosky, Breen, Graubard, & Parsons, 1998). Although individual patient characteristics are important, the characteristics of the examiner also play a significant role. A provider's specialty and age were identified in 1989 as significant predictors of physician adherence to the American Cancer Society's recommendations for rectal screening exams (Weisman, Celentano, Teitelbaum, & Klassen, 1989). Provider comfort, competence, and socioeconomic influences interact with the characteristics of the patient to influence the seeking and accepting of interventions.

According to Paglia (1999), "Male patients (are) more likely to . . . visit if their physician: did not (use) office assistance in matters of prevention, did not attempt a change in health behavior, learns about prevention through continuing medical education, and is a female geriatrician." Preceding and contradicting Paglia's finding, Morgan, Spencer, and King (1998) found that 84% of elderly had no preference as to whether the exam was performed by a female or male. But "female patients were more likely to . . . visit if their physician: did not have office assistance, was part of a group practice, and (the patient) had . . . a recent physical exam" (Paglia, 1999). And generally, men were more likely to have rectal exams and fecal occult blood testing (Borum, 1998). These recent studies support a different approach to male versus female elderly patients, an approach that is not necessarily politically correct, but definitely indicated by the research thus far.

Age, health care insurance, and sex are also important factors in the prevalence of anorectal exams. Recently documented, in a retrospective chart review of 200 ambulatory, internal medicine patients, at George Washington University Medical Center, patients age 50–60 had significantly more rectal examinations done than those 61–70 years (Borum, 1998). Essentially, the frequency of rectal exams declined significantly with age in this study, while colorectal cancer risk rose. Health care coverage, in addition to age, was identified as an important determinant of rectal screening exams in the 1992 National Health Interview Study (Potosky, Breen, Graubard, & Parsons, 1998). Interestingly, managed-care enrollees 65 years and older, were 10% more likely to be examined than elders enrolled in private, fee-for-service plans.

These are worrisome findings when we consider Morgan, Spencer, and King's 1998 study of 178 mentally alert elderly patients. Most (73%) of elders said they would feel "neutral," 13% "embarrassed," 11% "reluctant," and 2% "offended" if asked to submit to a rectal examination. Thirty-nine percent of the physicians, however, felt their elderly patients would be offended by the exam. Of the 76 general and geriatric physicians caring for the 178 patients in the study, only three said they would routinely do a rectal examination. Most of the elderly patients (76%) thought a rectal exam "important" and most seniors were willing to undergo examination if the physician asked. In another study (Morgan, Spencer, & King, 1998), of ten patients reported to physicians as fecally incontinent by nursing staff, only two had rectal exams. In spite of provider and patient apprehension, perianal and digital rectal exams are important, necessary components in the evaluation of perianal disease.

DEFINITIONS

Hemorrhoids

Often referred to as veins, hemorrhoids actually have an arterial pH and oxygen tension (Bilhartz & Croft, 2000), which produces bright red bleeding. Hemorrhoids, the vascular structures that line the rectal canal and the anal opening, are present episodically in virtually all patients. Internal hemorrhoids lie within the rectal vault, while external hemorrhoids are found at the anal verge. These vascular cushions may prolapse, thrombose, or incarcerate requiring surgical treatment. Prolapse, graded on a scale of one through four, usually precedes clot development and strangulation. Grade I describes the absence of prolapse, and Grade II is characterized by spontaneous reduction of the hemorrhoid after bowel movements. Grade III hemorrhoids require manual reduction of prolapse, and Grade IV is incarcerated. Gangrenous changes are possible in Grade IV hemorrhoids and require urgent surgical evaluation.

Rectal Prolapse

Often tolerated for years, rectal prolapse is a distressing condition characterized by the dropping or prolapse of the distal portion of the lower intestines. Detected by rectal exam, it is found in children and adults. There are three general types of rectal prolapse: complete prolapse, when the intestinal mucosa bulges through the anus, sometimes accompanied by peritoneal tissue and small bowel; concealed prolapse, when the upper rectum intussuscepts into the lower rectum but neither bulge through the anus; and incomplete prolapse, when a partial thickness of the intestinal wall drops or bulges inward (Andrew & Jones, 1992). Sometimes categorized as third-degree hemorrhoidal disease, the term anal prolapse is used in the European literature.

Rectal Masses

A mass in the rectum may signal hemorrhoids as previously discussed, impacted feces, abnormal prostate, genital warts, abscess, or cancer (Bilhartz & Croft, 2000). In the frail elderly, fecal impaction should be suspected and ruled out. Impaction of feces is an obstruction of the rectal vault by hardened stool, which generally occupies the complete volume of the distended rectum. Occasionally, in elderly men, prostate enlargement will encroach on the rectal cavity from the anterior wall of the distal colon. Generally seen perianally, condyloma acuminatum and rectal abscesses are due to infections of viral and bacterial pathogens respectively. Rectal cancer, usually the result of abnormal epithelial cell division, produces a space-occupying lesion, which is firm, fixed, and diagnosed by pathology after biopsy. While skin tags are considered benign, rectal polyps are generally viewed as precursors to rectal cancer.

ETIOLOGY

The incidence of lower gastrointestinal disease increases with age and is an important reason for medical visits (Chaplin, Curless, Thomson, & Barton, 2000). Constipation and lower urinary tract symptoms frequently occur in the elderly and some studies propose that dysfunction in one system may affect the other (Charach, Greenstein, Rabinovich, Groskopf, & Weintraub, 2001). In Charach and colleagues' study, 52 patients, aged 65 to 89 years, experienced significant improvement in quality of life, urinary symptoms, sexual function, and mood when their constipation was treated. Neurological disease, inactivity, and weak rectoperineal muscles have also been identified as likely causative factors of functional rectal disease in the elderly (Muller-Lissner, 2002). The affect of comorbidities, such as Parkinson's disease, should be considered when analyzing the contributing factors to anorectal disease. Anticholinergic medications, tricyclic antidepressants, opiates, oral iron preparations, anticonvulsants, and aluminum or calcium containing antacids can slow colonic transit times. With this plethora of influences, it is not surprising that seventy-one percent of examined elderly patients (Morgan, Spencer, & King, 1998) had positive findings on rectal exam. In all these cases the examination influenced treatment. Rectal mass, impacted feces, abnormal prostate, rectal prolapse, blood, and hemorrhoids were commonly detected. In this study, 61 of 178 patients were taking some type of laxative and only 22 had documented rectal exams.

Hemorrhoids

Frequent constipation and the use of laxatives have been commonly cited as causative in the development of hemorrhoids (Canadian Nursing Home Society, 1994). Current medical opinion cites fiber-poor foods, low fluid intake, inactivity, straining at stool and the normal senescence of the anorectal structures as significant antecedents (Guyton & Hall, 2001). Present in everyone at various times, hemorrhoids are prevalent, but not necessarily causative of many common anorectal symptoms.

Rectal Prolapse

Found in women six times more often than men, rectal prolapse is not caused by pregnancy or childbirth (Andrew & Jones, 1992). In the elderly, it is usually caused by constipation and straining at bowel movements. Prolapse may be spontaneous or occur with defecation, coughing, sneezing, or standing up. Usually reducible, rectal prolapse causes bleeding and mucosal discharge. Seventy-five percent of these patients have concomitant fecal incontinence.

Anorectal Masses

A rectal mass may be due to impacted feces, abnormal prostate, genital warts, abscess, or cancer. Fecal impaction is primarily caused by opioid medication use, dietary changes, prolonged inactivity, and chronic laxative use (Cefalu, McKnight, & Pike, 1981). Viruses, genes, radiation, and hormones are currently being investigated in the etiology of prostate cancer (National Cancer Institute, n.d.). Prostate volume is easily detected by palpation of the anterior rectal vault of male patients. A mass located anteriorly may represent prostate encroachment. Condyloma acuminatum is a highly infectious sexually transmitted disease caused by the human papilloma virus (HPV) and is believed to increase cancer risk (National Cancer, Institute, n.d.). Fleshy HPV anorectal growths may be visible perianally or palpable rectally. Infection can produce a tender rectal mass in the form of hidradenitis suppurativa, pilonidal disease, or solitary anorectal abscess (Bilhartz & Croft, 2000).

Rectal Cancer

Rectal cancer incidence peaks between 75 and 80 years old (Curless, French, Williams, & James, 1994). Rectal carcinogensis is multifactorial and our understanding of it is still evolving. While sedentary work, coffee or tea consumption, hormone replacement therapy, and nitrate exposure were identified as a risk factors for colon cancer, they have not been significant findings in etiological research on rectal cancer. Glycemic index, obesity, and fiber intake were identified as significant in a study (Franceschi, Dal Maso, Augustin, Negri, Parpinel, Boyle, et al., 2001). Exposure to the following substances "showed some association with rectal cancer: rubber dust, rubber pyrolysis products, cotton dust, wool fibers, rayon fibers, a group of solvents (carbon tetrachloride, methylene chloride, trichloroethylene, acetone, aliphatic ketones, aliphatic esters, toluene, styrene), polychloroprene, glass fibers, formaldehyde, extenders, and ionizing radiation" according to a case-control study by Dumas, Parent, Siemiatycki, and Brisson in Canada (2000). Ulcerative colitis, familial polyposis, past radiation therapy, viral infections, high iron with low vitamin C intake, beef intake, and alcohol use are all areas of current research related to rectal cancer risk (National Cancer Institute, n.d.).

Proctitis Ani

Commonly a symptom of infection or mechanical irritation, proctitis ani can also be a diagnosis of exclusion. Anal pruritis is a common complication after radiation therapy of the pelvic area and a frequent problem for hemorrhoid suffers. Infection and cancer can also produce perianal itching. It is important to exclude other causes before indulging in symptomatic management.

PATHOLOGY

The anus and rectal vault are together approximately 11 centimeters in length and distal to the colon. The rectum functions primarily in the storage of feces until the patient is able to defecate (Guyton & Hall, 2001). The anus, with its internal and external circular muscles, allows feces to pass the internal sphincter due to an involuntary relaxation triggered by the myenteric plexus. Defecation occurs only when the external anal sphincter is consciously relaxed at the same time peristalsis occurs. The intrinsic peristaltic reflex, however must be augmented by a "parasympathetic defecation reflex" for effective elimination, which is controlled by the sacral spinal cord (Guyton & Hall, 2001, p. 499). The sigmoid, rectal, and anal regions are richly innervated with parasympathetic nerve fibers. Sympathetic nervous system activity usually inhibits gastrointestinal as well as anorectal activity. Muscle stretching, stimulation by acetylcholine, activation of parasympathetic nerves, norepinephrine, or epinephrine can activate neural control of rectal smooth muscles.

Some research suggests there is a physiological decrease in rectal sensation with aging, which may explain elder symptomatology (Read, Abouzeki, & Read, 1985). Post mortem evaluation of the rectum across the life span reveals an increase in the amount of connective tissue to muscle tissue as patients age (Haas & Fox, 1980). Confined to the submucosal and subcutaneous layers, the shift in muscle to connective tissue ratio may have a role in the weakening of anal sphincters in the elderly. Slow colonic movement, pelvic dismotility, and increased rectal compliance were found by Merkel, Locher, Burgio, Towers, and Wald in their 1993 study of 18 chronic constipation suffers who were 60 years or older. Their research correlated physiological and psychological profiles in chronically constipated patients versus nonconstipated control subjects. One-third of these patients also had high scores of distress, somatization, depression, and anxiety on a self-rated inventory of psychological distress.

Hemorrhoids

The mean vascular pressure of rectal structures is about 17 to 25 mm Hg (Bilhartz & Croft, 2000). Lacking the continuous smooth muscle coat of the arterioles, these metarteriole structures are affected by the body's tissue metabolism, hydrostatic pressure, valve function, and arterial pressure pulsations. Vessels exposed to increased blood volume respond to the increased pressure with a stretching of the vessel walls. Dilated metarteriole vascular structures (internal hemorrhoids) are located in the hemorrhoidal columns on the left lateral, right anterior, and right posterior aspects of the rectal vault (Bilhartz & Croft, 2000). External hemorrhoids are located at the anal opening. Hemorrhoids are aggravated by valsalva maneuvers, which act as a tourniquet above the rectum causing blood pooling and distention of the vascular structures.

Rectal Prolapse

Frequently accompanied by fecal incontinence, patients with rectal prolapse commonly also have poor fixation of the rectum to the pelvis, a deep rectovaginal vault, deep rectovesical pouch, redundant colon, descending perineum, weak anal sphincter, and weak levator ani muscles (Andrew & Jones, 1992). It is unclear from the research at this time whether these factors are causal, secondary, or comorbid. Research shows constipation, hemorrhoids, and weak anal sphincters as frequent precursors to rectal prolapse, although the exact etiology is uncertain (Andrew & Jones, 1992). Probably starting as a concealed rectal prolapse of the upper rectum, the internal intussusception may progress to prolapse through the anus.

Medical treatments, while abundant, are considered variable in dependable outcome results. Historically, an encircling perianal suture was used on frail elderly who were unfit for surgery. This approach has fallen out of favor due to complications and poor functional outcomes. The Delorme procedure utilizes rectal mucosal excision then plication with sutures and currently provides a 67% improvement in continence (Kling, Rongione, Evans, & McFadden, 1996) and 5% recurrence rate (Ramanujam, Venkatesh, & Fietz, 1994). Laprascopic rectoplexy and/or perineal resection have been most successful in avoiding postoperative constipation and fecal leakage (Andrew & Jones, 1992).

Anorectal Masses

Fecal impaction is an obstruction of the anus or rectal vault by hardened stool. A frequent complication of chronic constipation in the elderly, fecal impaction commonly presents as overflow bowel incontinence (Prather & Borum, 2002), a failure of the patient to sense or act on the defecation urge. Common causes include mental impairment, decreased rectal sensation, and impaired rectopuborectal muscle function (Prather & Borum, 2002). In demented patients, fecal incontinence around the impaction may occur more frequently after eating due to activation of the gastrocolonic reflex.

Genital Warts

Described as a double-stranded DNA (deoxyribonucleic acid) virus, there are approximately 20 different types of HPV that cause genital warts. These small, pedunculated, cauliflower shaped, fleshy growths can affect the perianal or rectal canal. HPV types 16 and 18 are strongly associated with increased risk for anorectal cancer (National Cancer Institute, n.d.).

Commonly caused by staphylococci and streptococci organisms, hidradenitis suppurativa arises from sweat glands, pilonidal disease from hair follicles, and solitary anorectal abscesses from dermal tissue (Bilhartz & Croft, 2000).

Abnormal Prostate

Generally categorized into benign and malignant categories, prostate enlargement is common in men over 60 years of age. On rare occasions this structural enlargement can impede the movement of feces through the rectum. While not a focus of this discussion of anorectal disease, prostate enlargement should be considered when a firm mass is detected on the anterior wall of a male patient during DRE.

Rectal Cancer

Since colorectal cancer survival is affected by the stage of tumor growth at the time of diagnosis, delays in seeking medical care and age specific symptom clusters have been studied in the hope of improving treatment outcome. Rectal cancer patients typically present with local symptoms of tenesmus, abdominal pain, rectal pain, change in flatus production, and rectal mucous. Elderly patients are more likely to present with nonspecific gastrointestinal complaints, anorexia, falls, fatigue (Curless, French, Williams, & James, 1994) and anemia (Kemppainen, Raiha, Rajala, & Sourander, 1993).

Treatments are divided into surgical and medical approaches. Rectal cancers in elderly patients unsuitable for surgery are frequently treated effectively with radiation, bracytherapy, or chemotherapy and radiation (Schrag, Gelfand, Bach, Guillem, Minsky, & Begg, 2001). Some data suggests an increase of radiation sensitivity in the elderly due to reduced DNA repair mechanisms. However, research studies fail to prove radiation is less well tolerated by the elderly (Geinitz, Zimmerman, & Molls, 1999). More accurately stated, the elderly experience more functional mucositis, weight loss, and sexual dysfunction, as compared with younger patients who experience skin damage, nausea, and decreased pelvic radiotherapy effectiveness. In patients 65 years and older, surgery for rectal cancer has produced conflicting results of increased postoperative complications (Chippa, Zbar, Bertani, Audisio, & Staudacher, 2001) and morbidity/mortality comparable to younger patients (Puig-La, Quayle, Thaler, Shi, Paty, Quan, et al., 2000). Unfortunately, the medical treatment (radiation therapy) for various pelvic cancers can increase the risk of rectal bleeding in the aged and radiation induced rectal telangiectasias and bleeding have been documented (Niv & Henkin, 1995). Rectal ulcer has been identified as the cause of acute, painless, massive, fresh rectal bleeding in a study of three elderly bedridden patients over 80 years old (Takeuchi, Tsuzuki, Ando, Sekihara, Hara, Ohno, et al., 2001).

Proctitis Ani

Inflammation of the rectum is the general underlying mechanism for anal itching. Histamine, a powerful vasodilator, is released by mast cells into tissue when damage occurs (Guyton & Hall, 2001). Subsequent to histamine release, increased blood flow, edema, and itching occur. Rectal wall thickening and perirectal stranding has been identified in elders with systemic atherosclerosis (Bharucha, Tremaine, Johnson, & Batts, 1996). Acute ischemic proctosigmoiditis can occur with major hemodynamic illness. However, the incidence of ischemic proctolitis remains rare due to excellent collateral vessels in the rectal vault. Since innervation of the rectum is comparable in sensitivity to the fingertips, pruritis ani can be extremely disturbing.

GENERAL NURSING CARE

The American Nurses Association Standards of Clinical Nursing Practice guides our general nursing care of patients with anorectal problems. Utilizing nursing process, nursing care should provide culturally appropriate, age specific care; insure a safe environment; teach patients and family about interventions and health promotion activities; facilitate continuity of care; and communicate information effectively (American Nurses Association, 1998). The current research suggests that our biggest obstacle in caring for geriatric patients with anorectal disease is our omission of assessment for anal or rectal problems. Self-consciousness, apprehension, and personal aversion are best addressed through continuing education, mentorship, and self-reflection. Reassuringly, published articles on patient embarrassment, anger, fear, and complications related to nursing interventions are few and far between. Only one article, written in Israel and published in the United States, was found to contain a cautionary tale.

Infrequent, but important to avoid, is enema-induced perforation of the rectum with subsequent rectal bleeding (Paran, Butnaru, Neufeld, Magen, & Freund, 1999). Related to the enema tip or rectal tube retention balloon, these iatrogenic causes of rectal bleeding are more likely when a stricture, neoplasm, inflamed rectum, or history of prolonged steroid use is present (Williams & Harned, 1991). More frequently occurring in nursing homes, the chronically ill, and the chronically constipated, a diagnosis of rectal perforation is made by history, plain abdominal films, and CT scan. Fortunately, prompt diagnosis and surgical treatment insures a good outcome for the patient. Eight of the ten patients, in Paran and colleagues' (1999) study, presented to the emergency room with "vague and sometimes misleading" information from the nursing home.

The unique concerns of women and minorities are of special concern in the research, case finding, and treatment of anorectal disease, as in other diseases. Race continues to be a significant determinant of health in America and, unfortunately, the Latino, Black, and American Indian patient has been discriminated against, segregated, or exploited in research and treatment (McDonald, 1999). Policy barriers, health care provider ignorance, interpersonal communication difficulties, and racism have been identified. While researchers scramble to evaluate the impact and absence of minority and ethnic research data, nursing continues to embrace individualized patient advocacy from a holistic perspective.

Assessment

Theory-based nursing assessment begins with a patient history (Orem, 1995). A private setting, both visually and acoustically, insures the comfort of the examiner and patient. A focal assessment of the patient presenting with anemia of unknown origin is inappropriate due to the range of differential diagnoses. Patients who complain of signs or symptoms listed in Table 13.1, however should be questioned using Table 13.2. Historical assessment will include baseline bowel habits, analysis of symptoms, dietary practices, activity levels, educational level, primary language, source of health information (Yu, Kim, Chen, Brintnall, & Liu, 2001), and medication use.

Commonly presenting with anemia of unknown etiology, patients with rectal bleeding require a careful medical evaluation of the entire gastrointestinal system. In fact, blood loss was the most common presenting symptom found by Kemppainen, Raiha, Rajala, and Sourander (1993) in their study of 178 elderly colorectal patients. Additionally, there is a significant trend in the elderly toward underreporting of bowel habit change or rectal bleeding. The average delay in symptom reporting in the elderly is 19.5 weeks with a typical Dukes classification of C or worse at biopsy.

The physical exam, based on inspection and palpation techniques, follows the history and is best performed in a private room after patient consent. If done as a focal assessment, careful attention to patient teaching and consent is warranted. Examination begins with an explanation of the procedure and purpose of the exam. Nursing assistance may be helpful in the positioning and reassurance of the patient. Generally, the anorectal examination occurs after less embarrassing portions of the physical and, thus, falls into an expected flow of close scrutiny. For most patients, it is prudent and comforting when an abdominal evaluation is performed immediately prior to the anorectal exam.

Patients are most comfortable adequately covered and placed in the left lateral position (Bilhartz & Croft, 2000). Position the patient with buttocks slightly over the side of the bed or examining table. Care should be taken to insure the patient's safety and sense of security in the Sim's position. Gentle retraction of the superior buttock with the gloved right hand exposes the perianal area to inspection. The gloved left hand then lightly brushes the anal verge to elicit the "anal wink" reflex. Next produce mild traction at the anal margin to expose the distal anal lining. Finally, have the patient perform a brief valsalva maneuver to identify prolapse or fecal leakage. Salient findings in an anorectal examination are detailed in Table 13.3.

Digital rectal examination is an especially important part of the geriatric physical exam when anemia of unknown etiology is identified (Kemppainen, Raiha, Rajala, & Sourander, 1993), to rule out fecal impaction and to screen for prevalent rectal pathology (Morgan, Spencer, & King, 1998). In one study of 178 elders, 60% of all rectal cancers were identified by

TABLE 13.1   Common Signs & Symptoms of Anorectal Disease

Signs & Symptoms	
Bright red bleeding in streaks or drips	*Hemorrhoids*
Sensation of "protrusion"	
Pain with or without bowel movement:	
Burning	
Itching	
Lax anal tone	*Rectal prolapse*
Anus accommodates 2–3 fingers without pain	
Mucosa emerges through anus with straining	
Complete prolapse:	
Concentric folds of mucosa protrude from anus	
> 5 cm of mucosa	
Incomplete prolapse:	
Radial folds of mucosa with valsalva	
< 5 cm of mucosa	
Itching	
Feeling of incomplete defecation or protrusion	
Rarely bleeding	
Rectal cancer:	*Rectal mass*
Frequently occult blood or melena	
Obstipastion	
Occasionally blood mixed with stool	
Impacted feces:	
Fecal incontinence	
Abnormal prostate:	
Benign prostatic hypertrophy	
Prostate cancer	
Condyloma Acuminatum	
Pruritis	
Persistent "wetness"	
Serous discharge	
Scant bright red bleeding	
Occasional pain	
Occasional spotting of blood on toilet tissue	*Proctitis*
Mucus with stool	
Tenesmus	
Loose stools	
Gradually increasing throbbing pain	*Anorectal abscess*
Low grade fever	
Purulent drainage	

TABLE 13.2   Focal History-Taking in Anorectal Disease

Client Profile	Age, race, sex, marital status, religious orientation, educational level, language, occupation, family members/function, home and community characteristics, health goals? Initial determination of historical reliability
Universal self-care requisites	**Air:** Bathing practices, skin rash/pruritis/lesions, chills, SOB, dyspnea, palpitations, chest pain, orthopnea, cold extremities **Water:** Amount of daily fluid intake, fluid likes/dislikes, fluid temperature preferences, sweating, thirst, dry mouth, IVF, hyperalimentation **Food:** 24 diet recall (for daily fiber intake, 5 servings fruit/vegetables), food likes/dislikes, cultural/medical dietary modifications, food preparation, meal environment, access to fresh foods, food budgeting, food supplements, weight loss/gain, anorexia, indigestion, nausea, vomiting, prescribed or OTC medications, difficulties with teeth/gums/tongue/chewing, knowledge of food groups, current interest in changing dietary pattern on a scale of 1 to 10 **Elimination:** Last bowel movement, what frequency does patient consider normal, aware of bowel cues, frequency/consistency/ease/timing/color/odor/shape of bowel movements, recent changes in toileting routine, bowel aids, urinary incontinence, constipation, abdominal bloating, flatulence, rectal bleeding, pruritis, abdominal cramping, recent change in stool caliber/color, pain/pressure/appearance of masses with bowel movement, use of pads, # of underwear changes required **Activity and Rest:** Means of ambulation, difficulty (pain?) getting to water/fluid source, fear of falling, difficulty getting to toilet, level of activity, regular exercise, sleep/rest patterns, muscle weakness/tone, tremors, memory changes, avoids going out/changes in activity to avoid "accident" **Solitude and Social Interaction:** Mini Mental Status Exam, time/quality of time alone, time/quality of time with others, sexual practices, reproductive history, vision & hearing changes, social substance use (ETOH, drugs, coffee, tea, tobacco) use of health resources (last vaginal or digital rectal exam), locus of control (internal is positively correlated with seeking care), self concept, spiritual practices (fasting, food avoidance)

digital rectal exam (Kemppainen, Raiha, Rajala, & Sourander, 1993). However since nurses are not generally trained or licensed to detect anorectal disease, the initial rectal exam should be performed by a nurse practitioner or physician. Readily available in most patient care settings, the equipment necessary for a rectal exam includes disposable gloves and lubricating jelly.

TABLE 13.2 *(continued)*

Developmental self-care requisites	Life cycle stage: Freudian stage (psychosexual), Erikson stage (psychosocial), Piaget stage (intellectual), Kohlberg stage (moral); their effect on self-care knowledge/ability/results
Health deviation self-care requisites	**Current symptoms:** Gradual or sudden onset, alleviating/aggravating factors, occurs at night, episodic or chronic, associated with other symptoms, concerns about current symptoms (fear of incontinence), psychological/physical/financial effects of symptoms on life style, current/previous coping mechanisms, concurrent life stresses **Past Health Deviations:** Adult, childhood, accidents, hospitalizations, allergies, current & past medications, abdominal/pelvic surgeries **Family Health History**

While only 70–80% of the rectal vault mucosa can be palpated by the average examiner's finger, digital rectal exam (DRE) continues as a cornerstone of colorectal screening (Winawer & Shike, 1995). DRE carries neither risk of "false positives" found in fecal occult blood testing nor perforation risk (Mandel, Bond, & Church, 1993). In 1998, DRE was found to correlate strongly with anorectal manometry measures of anal sphincter function (Buch, Alos, Solana, Roig, Fernandez, & Diaz, 1998). Currently, the main limitation to screening effectiveness is the ability or willingness of patients and clinicians to comply with recommendations. Table 13.4 outlines current recommendations for DRE.

DRE should be performed slowly, with a lubricated gloved index finger, after telling the patient what to expect (Leffell, 1993). Begin by noting sphincter tone upon insertion and instruct the patient to squeeze. Palpate the circumference of the rectal vault above the anorectal ring by rotation of the examining finger. Anteriorly, the prostate in men and cervix in women may be noted. Extract the palpating finger and test the residual stool or mucus for occult blood. Reassure, drape, and notify the patient of the exam conclusion.

NURSING DIAGNOSES AND PLAN OF CARE

NANDA nursing diagnoses (Carpenito, 2002) for patients with anorectal disease are listed in Table 13.5. Considering the patient's basic, developmental, and health deviation aspects, Orem's (1995) holistic approach to

TABLE 13.3   Anorectal Inspection

Anatomical Area	Normal	Abnormal

Perianal skin	Intact
	Color consistent with race
		Blood
		Erosion
		Fissures
		Excoriation
		Masses:
		   Firm, fixed, nontender
		   Tender, firm or fluctuant
		   Multiple small furuncles
		   Tender, firm or fluctuant, upper gluteal cleft
		   Wart-like
		Scarring
		Erythema (or gray in Blacks)
		Rash
		Fistula
		Purulent discharge
		Pedunculated fleshy tags of skin
		Absent hair

Anal margin	Symmetrical anterior/ posterior margins	As above plus
		Mucosal folds:
		   Friable tissue
		   Radial folds
		   Concentric folds
		Red to bluish soft mass
		Erythematous firm tender mass
		Spasm

Distal rectal canal lining		As above plus Fissure or tear: White edges Pale, blue or black tissue Petechial hemorrhages Edema Fibrosis

self-care deficits facilitates identification of patient validated diagnoses. Culturally appropriate diagnosis and interventions are important to successful patient outcomes.

Outcome identification and collaborative goal setting should begin with human norms and the individual's history of bowel function. The range of normal bowel function varies from three bowel movements a day to one every three days (Bilhartz & Croft, 2000). Interim goals moving toward

TABLE 13.4   Current Recommendations for Rectal Exam

Organization	Start Age	Frequency	Exam Specifics
American Cancer Society 2001	50	Annual	DRE FOBT
American Gastroenterological Association 1997	50	Annual	FOBT
American Society for Gastrointestinal Endoscopy 1997	50	Annual	FOBT
American College of Colon and Rectal Surgeons 1999	50	Annual	FOBT
American College of Physicians 1997	50 if patient desires > 60 < 70	Annual	DRE FOBT
Institute for Clinical Systems Improvement 2001	> 50 < 80	Annual	FOBT
U.S. Preventive Services Task Force 2002	> 50	Annual	FOBT
American College of Preventive Medicine 1998	Recommends against routine screening		DRE

FOBT: fecal occult blood testing
DRE: digital rectal exam

the final outcome may be need to be considered. Patient abilities and limitations are frequently multifactorial in the control of anorectal function. Incremental progress can pose special challenges for the provider and patient but should be appreciated as necessary in some cases.

The educational aspects of anorectal nursing care are significant in number and complexity. Best prioritized in urgent nursing situations according to basic universal self-care requisites, long-term and less acute situations require incorporation and emphasis of developmental and health deviation requirements (see Table 13.2). The Nursing Outcomes Classification (NOC) domains of Functional, Physiological, Psychosocial, Knowledge, Behavior, and Perceived Health offer an assortment of Likert scale outcome measurements, which are useful in quantifying patient outcomes (Iowa Outcomes Project, 2000).

INTERVENTIONS, TREATMENTS, ALTERNATIVE TREATMENT

Serial anorectal assessment and traditional bowel training (adequate daily nutritional intake with fiber content appropriate for gender, height, and

TABLE 13.5   Alphabetical NANDA Nursing Diagnoses Related to Anorectal Disease

Activity Intolerance	Bowel Incontinence	Sleep Deprivation
Anxiety	Functional Incontinence	Disturbed Sleep Pattern
Impaired Bed Mobility	Reflex Incontinence	Impaired Social
Disturbed Body Image	Stress Incontinence	Interaction
Caregiver Role Strain	Total Incontinence	Social Isolation
Impaired Comfort	Urge Incontinence	Spiritual Distress
Confusion	Deficient Knowledge	Delayed Surgical
Constipation	Ineffective Therapeutic	Recovery
Perceived Constipation	Regimen Management	Disturbed Thought
Defensive Coping	Impaired Memory	Processes
Ineffective Coping	Imbalanced Nutrition:	Impaired Tissue Integrity
Altered Dentition	Less than Body	Impaired Urinary
Diarrhea	Requirements	Elimination
Dysreflexia	Pain	Urinary Retention
Adult Failure to Thrive	Impaired Physical	Impaired Walking
Risk for Falls	Mobility	Wandering
Fatigue	Post Trauma Syndrome	Impaired Wheelchair
Fluid Volume Deficit	Powerlessness	Mobility
Dysfunctional Grieving	Relocation Stress	Impaired Wheelchair
Impaired Health Mainten-	Self-care Deficit	Transfer Ability
ance	Syndrome	
	Self-care Deficit,	
	Toileting	
	Disturbed Self Concept	
	Disturbed Sensory	
	Perception	
	Impaired Skin Integrity	

weight; water intake of six to eight glasses daily; adequate daily exercises; nonrushed toileting on a planned schedule) are the cornerstones of elder nursing care. Traditional interventions are aimed at improving stool consistency, establishing an elimination routine, and stimulating predictable rectal emptying (International Foundation for Functional Gastrointestinal Disorders, 2002). Table 13.6 lists traditional generic nursing interventions commonly employed in anorectal care. Alternative or natural approaches to rectal function focus on diarrhea, constipation, and hemorrhoids.

Alternative Treatment

Excessive venous pressure is cited as causative in development of hemorrhoids by naturopathic physicians Shefrin, Pizzorno, and Murray (1999).

TABLE 13.6   Generic Nursing Interventions Specific to Anorectal Disease

Well-balanced, high-fiber meals:
  Include indigestible fiber such as whole grains, legumes, fresh fruits, and vegetables
  Gradually increase fiber up to 20 to 30 grams/day to avoid excess flatus

Assess readiness for training:
  Able to dress and undress self
  Able to understand and follow simple directions
  Takes pride in accomplishments
  Wants to put personal belongings where they belong
  Absence of significant negativity
  Bowel movements are well formed
  Able to remain clean for 2 hours at a time
  Aware of the need to eliminate
  Absence of restraints
  Mini Mental Status Exam

Agree on terms to be used by the patient and nurse for:
  Defecation
  Urgent rectal pressure
  Flatus
  Constipation
  Diarrhea
  Rectal leakage

Monitor for excessive flatulence, reduce the quantity of the following PRN:
  Raffinose—beans, cabbage, Brussels sprouts, broccoli, asparagus, whole grains
  Lactose—milk products (especially in African, Native American and Asian patients)
  Fructose—onions, artichokes, pears, wheat, soft drinks, fruit drinks
  Sucrose—apples, pears, peaches, prunes

Assess for:
  Anorectal incontinence
  Fecal impaction
  Rectal prolapse:
  Acute Strangulated—wrap with moist towels, urgent medical referral
  Chronic Episodic—bulk laxatives
  Incomplete—address fecal incontinence
  Signs and symptoms of anorectal disease

Provide regularly timed meals

8 glasses of water spaced over the day

Establish a regular time(s) for elimination:
  Morning
  20 to 30 minutes after a meal
  Benchmark against patient's baseline function and human norms

(continued)

TABLE 13.6 *(continued)*

Utilize the least noxious stimulus possible to promote elimination during training:
  Meal
  Hot drink
Manual disimpaction, suppository, enema, or laxative by nurse practitioner or physician
  Order

Maintain a Bowel Diary (Figure 13.1)

Maintain a Food Diary

Identify and accommodate patient mobility issues:
  Ambulation assistive devices
  Commode riser
  Commode handrails
  Transfer techniques
  Bedside commode
  Distance to bathroom
  Vision correction

Identify, modify, or accommodate environmental barriers:
  Adequate lighting
  Privacy
  Remove throw rugs
  Handrails
  Supplies within reach of the toilet
  Ramps versus stairs
  Clear, short path to bathroom
  Adequate bathroom space for walker, cane, or wheelchair

Teach pelvic floor exercises

Reinforce t.i.d. practice of pelvic floor exercises

If lack of progress consider:
  Repeating readiness assessment
  The point at which progress ceased and contributing factors
  Biofeedback training—neuromuscular retraining with sensors and graphs
  Anal manometry-anorectal pressures
  Endoanal ultrasound
  Endoscopy
  Electromyography
  Defacatography—evaluation of rectal and anal function
  Neosphincter reconstruction

TABLE 13.6 (*continued*)

Postoperative sphincteroplasty care

Assess for common aggravating factors:
  Diarrhea
  Psoriasis
  Eczema
  Yeast
  Coffee intake
  Citrus fruits
  Antibiotics

Teach gentle post-defecation cleansing methods:
  Avoid furious wiping with dry toilet paper
  Avoid leaving residual bits of toilet paper on the perianal skin after cleansing
  Avoid dyes, perfumes, and colors in toilet paper
  Use warm water only to avoid stripping skin of natural protection
  Limit sitz baths to a couple of minutes when used for cleansing purposes
  Dry the skin thoroughly by patting dry or use a fan
  Cleanse after exercise and long periods of sitting
  Wash hands after elimination

Avoid potentially irritating over the counter products containing:
  Anesthetics
  Witch hazel
  Alcohol

When using ointments, use a thin layer to avoid:
  Interfering with anal closure
  Trapping bacteria, yeast or fungus against delicate perianal skin

Non-medicated talcum powder or cornstarch may be used to dry and sooth skin

A mild acid-based cortisone cream may be prescribed and utilized briefly to break the
  itch-scratch cycle

Underclothes should be:
  Loose
  Dye free
  Washed in non-allergenic soap

Avoid sitting for long periods
  Consider use of a "donut shaped cushion" to reduce skin pressure

Odor control:
  Environmental sprays
  Airtight dirty linen storage
  Prompt clothing and linen changes
  Chlorophyllin—oral or topical, green staining of body fluids may occur
  Charcoal—oral

(continued)

TABLE 13.6 *(continued)*

General education—Explain, document and reinforce:
  Disease risk, pathophysiology, care plan, outcome measures, collaborative goals, potential benefits & complication risks of testing/treatment, probability of "false positives"
  and the nature of follow up testing if an abnormality is identified, routine follow-
  up recommendations

Common sources of increased intra-abdominal pressure include: defecation, pregnancy, coughing, sneezing, vomiting, physical exertion, and
standing or sitting for prolonged periods. These sources of increased pressure are targeted for intervention, along with dietary fiber, yeast overgrowth, parasitic infections, and allergen elimination. Interestingly,
traditional medicine's frequent omission of anorectal examination is well
known in alternative medicine circles (Shefrin, Pizzorno, & Murray, 1999).
Natural and allopathic therapies are contrasted in Table 13.7. In both types
of medicine, nutritional approaches are foundational, and typically try the
least invasive interventions progressively before surgical options are
recommended.

HEALTH PROMOTION AND QUALITY OF LIFE ISSUES

Health promotion and disease prevention in older adults is evolving but
general agreement exists on its importance (Paglia, 1999). Prevention of
anorectal disease involves a proactive lifelong approach to elimination. It
is not unrealistic to say this approach begins with childhood toilet training.
Individual experiences, parental interactions, and behavioral training methods related to anal rectal function vary tremendously. So profound are
their effects that Freud identified toilet training as a crucial step in the
individual's psychosexual development. The time taken to explore and
analyze each patient's experience of this developmental stage can yield
significant insight toward developing a wellness diagnosis. Inherent in
nursing care for health promotion is the identification of patterns of wellness, healthy responses, and client abilities (Carpenito, 2002).
   A soft, bulky stool, passed with ease daily to every third day, is the
standard for rectal health. Tables 13.1, 13.2, 13.3, and 13.6 provide detailed
assessment points which provide important information on coping skills
and the absence or control of symptoms. The Bowel Diary (Fig. 13.1) can

TABLE 13.7 Hemorrhoid Treatments in Natural Medicine and Allopathic Medicine

	Natural Medicine	Allopathic Medicine
Nutrition	High-fiber, high-carbohydrate diet which includes liberal amounts of: Blackberries Cherries Blueberries Garlic Onions Ginger Cayenne 5 servings/day of fruits/vegetables Always eat breakfast (Klenner, 1971) Eliminate obesity	High-fiber diet: 25 grams/day 6–8 glasses of water/day
Topical	Witch hazel compress (Hamamelis Virginiana) Essential oils: Shark liver, cod liver, almond, cypress, juniper, lavender, lavender, lemon, rosemary Aloe vera gel Cocoa butter Peruvian balsam Zinc oxide Live yeast derivative Poultice/paste: Plantain from plantago Aesculus hippocastanum Comfrey and vegetable oil Calendula Chamomile Yarrow Ruscus aculeatus tincture Tea for topical application: Alumroot, goldenseal, mullein, slippery elm bark	Over-the-counter treatments not proven effective, not recommended but not discouraged
Hydrotherapy	Sitz bath (hot sitz bath* 3–10 minutes at 105–115 degrees F at a level at least 1 inch above the level used for the following cold sitz bath of 1–3 minutes at 55–75 degrees F, *accompanied with hot foot bath)	

(continued)

TABLE 13.7 (*continued*)

	Natural Medicine	Allopathic Medicine
Supplements	Psyllium seed and guar gum fiber, 4–10 teaspoons/day Citrus bioflavonoids: (Hydroxyethylrutosides) Vitamin A 10, 000 IU/day Vitamin B-complex 10–100 mg/day Vitamin C 500–3,000 mg/day Vitamin E 200–600 IU/day Bioflavinoids 100–1,000 mg/day Zinc 15–30 mg/day	
Medicines	Centella asiatica extract, 70% triterpenic acid content, 30 mg t.i.d, p.o. Aesculus hippocastanum bark of root, 500 mg t.i.d, p.o. Ruscus aculeatus, 9–11% ruscogenin content, 100 mg t.i.d, p.o. Aloe vera powder laxative 0.05–0.2 gram	Stool softener for 4 weeks
Activity	Regular exercise Avoid prolonged standing in one place Never ignore "the urge to go" Relax when sitting on the toilet Don't sit on the toilet longer than necessary Adopt more of a squatting position on the toilet: raise your feet on a small step stool	
Surgical	Sclerosing agents Rubber band ligation Cryosurgery Hemorroidectomy Infrared coagulation Direct current cautery	Excision Sclerosing agents Rubber band ligation

be used to collect and quantify anorectal function at any time. Frequently, additional health benefits are conferred in the wellness interaction through the nurse-patient relationship. The therapeutic effects of interpersonal rapport, compassion for the individual, satisfaction at being understood, receiving empathy, and confidentiality experienced by the patient can be profound.

Document three codes in each block based on the codes listed below.

	Sunday	Monday	Tuesday	Wednesday	Thursday	Friday	Saturday
Wake up toilet							
Morning toilet							
6 a - 9 a							
9 a - 12 n							
12 n - 3 p							
3 p - 6 p							
6 p - 9 p							
Bedtime toilet							
Awaken from sleep							
Comments							

Results code: C—Continent stool; SS—Slightly soiling; S—Staining
Description of feces: F—Formed stool; L—Loose stool; W—Watery stool
Aware of "urge to go": Y—yes, N—no

FIGURE 13.1 Bowel diary.

Annual assessment, examination, and education are important to elder health promotion and quality of life (Yu, Kim, Chen, Brintnall, & Liu, 2001). Fortunately, Medicare Part B covers annual colorectal preventive screening. Quality of life in the aged requires the assessment dimensions of physical, psychological, social, spiritual, support systems, symptoms, and functional aspects. The measurement of these dimensions yields a determination of patient well-being, meaning, and value (Sarvimaki & Stenbock-Hult, 2000). Annual patient interactions should include education and reinforcement of disease risk, warning signs, and instructions on seeking appropriate care. Empowerment through knowledge of symptom reporting, effective symptom management, and likely treatment outcomes serves to increase older adults' self-confidence and sense of well-being. Table 13.8 identifies common nursing diagnoses in positive anorectal function.

HOME MANAGEMENT AND SELF-CARE ISSUES

Most interventions for rectal and anal symptoms listed in Table 13.6 are easily used in the home environment. Soothing astringent and vasoactive medicines can be purchased at drug, department, and natural food stores throughout the country. The durable medical equipment required is generally available from local medical supply stores, classified newspaper ads, or flea markets. Insurance reimbursement varies widely by plan and should be explored thoroughly at the time medical necessity develops. Area disease-specific nonprofit organizations, spiritually based outreach programs, and government-sponsored resources for the aged are all legitimate sources of patient support.

TABLE 13.8 Wellness Nursing Diagnoses Related to Anorectal Disease

Positive Health Perception
Effective Health Management
Effective Nutritional-Metabolic Pattern
Effective Activity-Exercise Pattern
Effective Sleep-Rest Pattern
Positive Cognitive-Perception Pattern
Positive Self-Perception Pattern
Effective Coping-Stress Tolerance Pattern
Positive Value-Belief Pattern

Patient self-care may require the complete or partial assistance of family or friends, and everyone involved should remain sensitive to the fact that these issues are delicate and potentially embarrassing to the patient and his or her family. The patient's willingness, manipulative skills, and sensory and reasoning abilities will influence the need for assistance. Resistance to physical care is common in demented patients and therefore offers unique challenges to healthcare providers (Stewart, Gonzalez-Perez, & Zhu, 1999). Make every effort to anticipate needed caregiver assistance for the patient's specific plan of care. Demonstration of self-care activities by the patient is an especially good method of confirming the amount of assistance needed. Family or friends who are uncomfortable with direct patient care activities can help with transportation, financial assistance with supplies, home environmental modifications, companionship, and reassurance.

FOLLOW-UP CARE

Due to the high frequency of colorectal and prostate disease, annual rectal examinations, stool analysis for guaiac, and a high index of suspicion are recommended (Robie, 1989). Disease-specific medical follow-up is generally monthly during treatment of nonemergency anorectal problems. Routine nursing care frequency is determined through nurse-patient collaborative goal setting and NOC selection.

REFERENCES

Andrew, N. J., & Jones, D. J. (1992). Rectal prolapse and associated conditions. *British Medical Journal, 305*(6847), 234.

American Nurses Association (1998). *Standards of Clinical Nursing Practice* (2nd ed.). Washington, DC: Author.

Bharucha, A. E., Tremaine, W. J., Johnson, C. D., & Batts, K. P. (1996). Ischemic proctosigmoiditis. *American Journal of Gastroenterology, 91*(11), 2305–2309.

Bilhartz, L. E., & Croft, C. L. (2000). *Gastrointestinal disease in primary care.* Philadelphia: Lippincott Williams & Wilkins.

Borum, M. L. (1998). Does age influence screening for colorectal cancer? *Age and Aging, 27*(4), 508.

Buch, E., Alos, R., Solana, A., Roig, J. V., Fernandez, C., & Diaz, F. (1998). Can digital examination substitute anorectal manometry for the evaluation of anal canal pressures? *Revista Espanola de Enfermedades Digestivas, 90*(2), 90–93.

Canadian Nursing Home Society. (1994). Managing hemorrhoids. *Canadian Nursing Home, May–June, 5*(2), 26–27.

Carpenito, L. J. (2002). *Nursing diagnosis: Application to clinical practice.* Philadelphia: Lippincott.

Cefalu, C. A., McKnight, G. T., & Pike, J. I. (1981). Treating impaction: A practical approach to an unpleasant problem. *Geriatrics, 36*(5), 143–146.

Chaplin, A., Curless, R., Thomson, R., & Barton, R. (2000). Prevalence of lower gastrointestinal symptoms and associated consultation behaviour in a British elderly population determined by face-to-face interview. *British Journal of General Practice, 50*(459), 798–802.

Charach, G., Greenstein, A., Rabinovich, P., Groskopf, I., & Weintraub, M. (2001). Alleviating constipation in the elderly improves urinary tract symptoms. *Gerontology, 47*(2), 72–76.

Chippa, A., Zbar, A. P., Bertani, E., Biella, F., Audisio, R. A., & Staudacher, C. (2001). Surgical outcomes for colorectal cancer patients including the elderly. *Hepato-gastroenterology, 48*(38), 440–444.

Curless, R., French, J. M., Williams, G. V., & James, O. J. (1994). Colorectal carcinoma: Do elderly patients present differently? *Age and Aging, 23*(2), 102.

Dumas, S., Parent, M. E., Siemiatycki, J., & Brisson, J. (2000). Rectal cancer and occupational risk factors: A hypothesis-generating, exposure-based case control study. *International Journal of Cancer, 87*(6), 874–879.

Franceschi, S., Dal Maso, L., Augustin, L., Negri, E., Parpinel, M., Boyle, P., Jenkins, D. J., & LaVecchia, C. (2001). Dietary glycemic load and colorectal cancer risk. *Annals of Oncology: Official Journal of the European Society for Medical Oncology, 12*(2), 173–178.

Geinitz, H., Zimmerman, F. B., & Molls, M. (1999). Radiotherapy of elderly patients. *Organ der Deutschen Roentgengesellschaft, 175*(3), 119–127.

Guyton, A. C., & Hall, J. E. (2001). *Textbook of medical physiology* (10th ed). Philadelphia: W. B. Saunders Company.

Haas, P. A., & Fox, T. A. (1980). Age-related changes and scar formations of perianal connective tissue. *Disease of the Colon and Rectum, 23*(3), 160–169.

Iowa Outcomes Project (2000). In M. Johnson, M. Maas, & S. Moorehead (Eds.), *Nursing outcomes classification* (2nd ed). St. Louis: Mosby, Inc.

International Foundation for Functional Gastrointestinal Disorders (2002). Retrieved July 28, 2002 from *http://www.aboutincontinence.org/BowelControl.html*

Kemppainen, M., Raiha, I., Rajala, T., & Sourander, L. (1993). Delay in diagnosis of colorectal cancer in elderly patients. *Age and Aging, 22*(4), 260.

Kling, K. M., Rongione, A. J., Evans, B., & McFadden, D. W. (1996). The Delorme procedure: A useful operation for complicated rectal prolapse in the elderly. *American Surgeon, 62*(10), 857–860.

Leffell, D. J. (1993). The effect of pre-education on patient compliance with full body examination in a public skin cancer screening. *Journal of Dermatological Surgery and Oncology, 19*(7), 660–663.

Mandel, J. S., Bond, J. H., & Chursch, T. R. (1993). Reducing mortality from colorectal cancer by screening for fecal occult blood. *New England Journal of Medicine, 332,* 1365–1371.

McDonald, C. (1999). Cancer statistics: Challenges in minority populations. *A Cancer Journal for Clinicians, 49*(1), 6–7.

Merkel, I. S., Locher, J., Burgio, K., Towers, A., & Wald, A. (1993). Physiologic and psychologic characteristics of an elderly population with chronic constipation. *American Journal of Gastroenterology, 88*(11), 1854–1859.

Morgan, R., Spencer, B., & King, D. (1998). Rectal examination in elderly subjects: Attitudes of patients and doctors. *Age and Aging, 27*(3), 353.

Muller-Lissner, S. (2002). General geriatrics and gastroenterology: Constipation and fecal incontinence. *Clinical Gastroenterology, 16*(1), 115–133.

National Cancer Institute (n.d.). Cancer research portfolio. Retrieved July 28, 2002 from *http://researchportfolio.cancer.gov/*

Niv, Y., & Henkin, Y. (1995). *Journal of Clinical Gastroenterology, 21*(4), 295–297.

Orem, D. E. (1995). *Nursing: Concepts of practice.* St. Louis: Mosby, Inc.

Paglia, M. J. (1999). Dissertation Abstracts International: Section B. *The Sciences & Engineering, 60*(2-B), 0606.

Paran, H., Butnaru, G., Neufeld, D., Magen, A., & Freund, U. (1999). Enema-induced perforation of the rectum in chronically constipated patients. *Diseases of the Colon and Rectum, 42*(12), 1609–1612.

Potosky, A. L., Breen, N., Graubard, B. I., & Parsons, P. E. (1998). The association between health care coverage and the use of cancer screening tests: Results from the 1992 National Health Interview Survey. *Medical Care, 36*(3), 257–270.

Prather, C., & Borum, M. (2002). Constipation, diarrhea and fecal incontinence. Retrieved June 28, 2002 from *http://www.merck.com/pubs/mm_geriatrics/sec13/ch110.htm*

Puig-La, J., Quayle, J., Thaler, H. T., Shi, W., Paty, P. B., Quan, S. H., Cohen, A. M., & Guillem, J. G. (2000). Favorable short-term and long-term outcome after elective radical rectal cancer resection in patients 75 years of age or older. *Diseases of the Colon and Rectum, 43*(12), 1704–1709.

Ramanujam, P. S., Venkatesh, K. S., & Fietz, M. J. (1994). Perineal excision of rectal procidentia in elderly high-risk patients. *Diseases of the Colon and Rectum, 37*(10), 1027–1030.

Read, N. W., Abouzeki, L., & Read, M. G. (1985). Anorectal function in elderly patients with fecal impaction. *Gastroenterology, 89,* 959–966.

Robie, P. W. (1989). Cancer screening in the elderly. *Journal of the American Geriatrics Society, 37*(9), 888–893.

Sarvimaki, A., & Stenbock-Hult, B. (2000). Quality of life in old age described as a sense of well-being, meaning and value. *Journal of Advanced Nursing, 32*(4), 1025–1033.

Schrag, D., Gelfand, S. E., Bach, P. B., Guillem, J., Minsky, B. D., & Begg, C. B. (2001). Who gets adjuvant treatment for stage II and III rectal cancer? *Journal of Clinical Oncology, 19*(17), 3712–3718.

Shefrin, D. K., Pizzorno, J. E., & Murray, M. T. (Eds.) (1999). *Textbook of natural medicine* (2nd ed.). Edinburgh: Churchill Livingstone.

Stewart, J. T., Gonzalez-Perez, E., & Zhu, Y. (1999). Resistiveness to physical care. *American Journal of Geriatric Psychiatry, 7*(3), 259–263.

Takeuchi, K., Tsuzuki, Y., Ando, T., Sekihara, M., Hara, T., Ohno, Y., Yoshikawa, M., & Kuwano, H. (2001). Clinical characteristics of acute hemorrhagic rectal ulcer. *Journal of Clinical Gastroenterology, 33*(3), 226–228.

Weisman, C. S., Celentano, D. D., Teitelbaum, M. A., & Klassen, A. C. (1989). Cancer screening services in the elderly. *Public Health Reports, 104*(3), 209–214.

Williams, S. M., & Harned, R. K. (1991). Recognition and prevention of barium enema complications. *Current Problems in Diagnostic Radiology, 20*(4), 123–151.

Winawer, S. J., & Shike, M. (1995). Prevention and control of colorectal cancer. In P. Greenwald, B. S. Kramer, & D. L. Weed (Eds.), *Cancer prevention and control.* New York: Marcel Dekker.

Yu, E. S. H., Kim, K. K., Chen, E. H., Brintnall, R. A., & Liu, W. T. (2001). Colorectal cancer screening among Chinese Americans: A community-based study of knowledge and practice. *Journal of Psychosocial Oncology, 19*(3–4), 97–112.

Index

Springer Publishing Company

Physical Change and Aging, *4th Edition*
A Guide for the Helping Professions
Sue V. Saxon, PhD, Mary Jean Etten, EdD, GNP

The physical changes and the common pathologies associated with aging are discussed, along with the psychological and social implications of such changes. The guide is for nurses, gerontologists, social workers, psychologists, rehabilitation specialists and others in the helping professions.

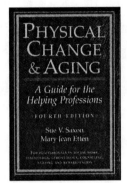

Partial Contents:

- Perspectives on Aging
- Theories on Aging
- Skin, Hair, and Nails
- The Musculoskeletal System
- The Nervous Systems
- Dementia and Delirium
- The Sensory System
- The Cardiovascular System
- The Respiratory System
- The Gastrointestinal System
- The Urinary System
- The Reproductive System
- The Endocrine System
- The Immune System
- Health Promotion and Exercise
- Nutrition
- Medication and the Elderly

2002   0-8261-1655-8   480pp   softcover
Originally published by The Tiresias Press, Inc.

536 Broadway, New York, NY 10012
Order Toll-Free: 877-687-7476 • Order On-line: www.springerpub.com

Springer Publishing Company

The Encyclopedia of Elder Care
The Comprehensive Resource on Geriatric and Social Care

Mathy D. Mezey, RN, EdD, FAAN, Editor-in-Chief
Barbara J. Berkman, DSW, **Christopher M. Callahan,** MD,
Terry Fulmer, RN, PhD, FAAN, **Gregory J. Paveza,** MSW, PhD, ACSW,
Eugenia L. Siegler, MD, and **Neville E. Strumpf,** PhD, RN, FAAN, Associate Editors
Melissa M. Bottrell, MPH, Managing Editor

"...The Encyclopedia of Elder Care *provides a wealth of up-to-date, well-referenced coverage of clinical subjects related to the older adult."*
—**Contemporary Gerontology**

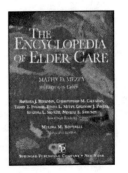

Focusing on the broad but practical notions of how to care for the patient, *The Encyclopedia of Elder Care,* a state-of-the-art resource, features nearly 300 articles written by experts in the field. Multidisciplinary by nature, all aspects of clinical care of the elderly are addressed. Each article concludes with specialty Website listings to help direct the reader to further resources.

A first in the field, *The Encyclopedia* will prove to be an indispensable tool for all professionals in the field of aging.

Topics covered include the following:

- Chronic Illness
- Consumer Directed Care
- Dementia
- Exercise and the Cardiovascular Response
- Fractures
- Glaucoma
- Hearing Impairment
- Infection Transmission in Institutions
- Joint Replacement
- Nutritional Assessment
- Over-the-Counter Drugs and Self-Medication
- Pain
- Psychological/Mental Status Assessment
- Quality of Life Assessment
- Respite Care
- Self Care
- Sexual Health
- Social Supports
- Stroke
- Swallowing Disorders
- Urinary Incontinence
- Weakness

2001   824pp   0-8261-1368-0   hardcover

536 Broadway, New York, NY 10012
Order Toll-Free: 877-687-7476 • Order On-line: www.springerpub.com